Adolescents and Soci... g

Javed Khan

TABLE OF CONTENTS

CHAPTER NO.	TITLE	PAGE NO.

CHAPTER NO.	TITLE	PAGE NO.

CHAPTER NO.	TITLE	PAGE NO.

CHAPTER NO.	TITLE	PAGE NO.

CHAPTER NO.	TITLE	PAGE NO.

CHAPTER NO.	TITLE	PAGE NO.

CHAPTER 1

INTRODUCTION

1.1 INTRODUCTION

In the century we live in, the digital epoch, social networking has gained enormously vital momentum in human life and it has an outstanding role in this picture. The electronic communication revolution plays a task in bridging the gap connecting the developed and developing countries; the rich and the poor. Irrespective of caste, creed, color, sex, young / old, professionals and homemakers alike are immersed in social networking and it has become inextricable. As per Itu, I. T. U. (2018), 80.9% of the natives in developed countries and 41.1% of citizens in developing countries used the internet in 2017. In the year 2019, the number of internet users globally is 4.388 billion. As of January 2019; the lively internet users are around 4.4 billion, which is parallel to 57% of the global population (Hoot Suite Digital 2019). In 2021 in India, 624 million (45%) citizens access internet, 572 million people use mobile to access internet and out of them 444 million are social networking users whereas; 66.6% of the people in the globe make use of a mobile phone, 4.66 billion utilize internet and 4.20 billion access social networking (Social, W. A. 2020).

Social networking has emerged to be an authoritative tool of communication. Online activity has become detrimental for everyone to interfere with daily life. This has become a comprehensive occurrence and a central means of relationship within the families, friends, classmates, and colleagues. The level of fame and social networking has augmented to a great extent over the years. A chief path for every day social communication is created because of the ease of use and access to broadband / mobile data facilities, rise in the figure of social networking along with the swift augmentation and encroachment of technology in the recent years. Various purpose of engaging in it is to have fun, to gain knowledge, to interact with others and to shop online. Naslund, J. A., (2016) mentioned that virtual communities, allows client to connect with other individuals based on familiar interests to share out, co-create or switch over information, data, videos, photos etc. People also employ in quite a lot of deeds on it, an extremely enlightening and amusing medium as per Kuss, D. J., & Griffiths, M. D. (2011); in short one can access social networking for education, entertainment, communication and information-sharing.

In the Indian scenario, the internet is conquered by the necessity to converse and socialize with others. India is on its means to achieve a position as a digitally advanced nation, a dwelling place to one of the world's prime, swiftly mounting digital clients. Internet and Mobile Association of India, reports that the existing figures of people using internet in India is 300 million. Economic Times Bureau (2016), Internet and Mobile Association of India (2015) reports that 80% of Internet users from Urban India used the Internet for online communication, 74% for social networking, 30% for enjoyment, 13% online shopping, and 11% for buying online tickets. According to Kuss, D. J., & Griffiths, M. D. (2011) Indian citizens waste extra time in social networking, more than China and the United States; that is 17 hours in every week.

In India, adolescents squander most of their leisure time by simply surfing the internet, ogling their smart phone and satisfy their needs through this, instead of spending time with their loved ones, finally they will be out from the actual world because of the constant use. They start yearning for gadget and social networking in the absence of it and some land up in unscrupulous activities. Increased social networking can lead to physical, academic, psychological, adjustment and familial impacts. Distractions from studies occur due to the involvement in social networking, as the adolescents pay more attention in it, can have a detrimental bang on the academics and can lead to academic failure.

The negative impacts of social networking can slither the adolescents into addiction. Generally people think that addiction occur due to psycho active substance use such as alcohol. Unmanageable practices or behavior is also referred to as addiction (Harris, P., et al 2014). Raj, M., et al (2018) reported that the time spend in social networking is related to addiction, the more they spend time in it more will be the addiction. The behavior of excessive and unnecessary engagement in social networking leading to development of addiction has become a major issue in a swiftly mounting country like India. In reality, it is not an exaggeration if we say that, social networking is an extensively used means to foster addictive behavior among adolescents.

A major concern is that this addictive behavior can reduce the mental health of the adolescents. Recent studies by Abi-Jaoude, E., et al (2020) found that social networking addiction can lead to fluctuations in the mood / sleep, suicidal ideations and poor mental health (Balcerowska, J. M., et al 2020). Thus stress, anxiety and depression arise because of social networking addiction (Saikia et al 2019).

1.2 NEED FOR THE STUDY

In India, social networking research is in its formative years, as such the social networking addiction and its related issues need further exploration. India is embracing technological intensification at a pace faster than ever, there is a nation-wide call for action to conduct robust researches to support the influence of social networking on mental health and to generate alertness on planning public health policies with regard to this addiction.

It is a fact that the interaction and communication of adolescents can be improved through social networking. It helps in making new friends, swaps over ideas and pictures, helps in building new interests and enhances self-expression. The fundamental skills in social and technical area are learnt through social networking, which are considered to be vital to survive in the modern society. An adolescent with trouble in building contacts, difficulty in maintaining face to face interaction will establish relation with others and will have a huge pack of friends in social networking. Moreover, the time adolescents fritter in front of the gadgets has increased with the boost in the figure of social networking sites. As a result of this, face to face communication will reduce further and there is more chance of escaping from their real life responsibilities.

Globally, 3.8% of the adolescents report severe mental health problems such as depression (World Health Organization 2011). 7.5% have one or the other mental illness, depression is noted in 56 million and anxiety in 38 million Indians. It was estimated that by the end of 2020, 20 per cent of Indian citizens will suffer from mental illnesses (World Health Organization 2020). As far as the Indian context is concerned, 14-40% of adolescents were assumed to have mental health problems related to internet addiction. Arumugam, B., et al (2014) stated that this addiction might possibly have bad effect on the fitness of the users. Physical effects include involvement of brain, hearing, vision, bone, muscles and heart. Psychological effects include anxiety, disturbed sleep pattern, fatigue, loneliness and depression. Social problems include academic turn down, relationship problems, and social isolation (Chou, C., et al 2005); reduced subjective well-being increases features of depression (Kross, E., et al 2013).

(Young, K. S., & Rogers, R. C. 1998; Nalwa, K., & Anand, A. P. 2003; Widyanto, L., & Griffiths, M. 2006; Christakis, D. A., et al 2011); reported that student population is mainly prone for using the internet excessively as they depend upon it for their instructive needs. This pushes more and more students towards escalating dependence on the internet. Ultimately they switch from the instructional use to the unhealthy use. Thus the lengthy engagement in social networking among adolescents can root negative outcomes such as mounting contact to strangers, cyber-bullying, online dating, decreased sleep, contact to incongruous content, poor social interactions and limited face to face communication.

Adolescents base their online fame on the figure of "friends" or "followers" they have in social networking sites causing them to get into a crazy chase to increase this number. Valkenburg, P. M., et al (2006) stated that social networking is a straight signal of insecurity and low self-esteem, a dependence on reassurance from others in the form of "likes" or complements, since they are deficient in self-confidence in the real world. The cause of social networking addiction chiefly at some point in adolescence consist of their demand to get pleasure from autonomy, yearning to accomplish dominance, to execute their fantasies, to break out of family and to avoid emotional breakdown. The quintessence of the social networking is that it attracts the user to itself by activating the reward system in the brain that causes the individual to keep returning to it.

Internet addiction disorder (IAD) is common among adolescents. It is the inability to control internet usage that can result in physical, psychological and social problems; features include salience, mood modification, tolerance, withdrawal symptoms, conflict and relapse (Young, K. S., & Rogers, R. C. 1998). Individuals who are prone for internet addiction will be generally uncomfortable and are often insecure about their relationships with others. They fear refusal and aloneness due to supposed incapability to stimulate the attention of others in real life. This causes them to go round to the internet where they discover reception from like-minded individuals. Social networking addiction can have harmful effect on adolescents, the stimulation outline which occurs in social networking addiction is similar to other addictions.

Today's adolescents are tomorrow's citizens; mentally healthy adolescents will contribute positively to the productivity of the nation. Adolescents show a passionate curiosity in social networking at this stage. The widespread exploit of social networking in India has been on the mount among them. At this time, they fall into addiction due to peer pressure, craziness, revolt against someone / something, or to mimic adults. It is significant to investigate the influence of social networking on mental health among adolescents and no researcher has appropriately selected this area of research.

1.3 STATEMENT OF PROBLEM

As far as the adolescents are concerned, they are in the transition phase and will be stressed because of various reasons. They are more interested in mingling with friends and moreover engrossed towards electronic gadgets. Moreover the adolescents prefer to be independent and like privacy; which they find from social networking. The diverse features and tendency to explore social networking increases the usage. Even though the adolescents start engaging in social networking for academic purpose, gradually the intention can change, increased intensity can lead to negative impacts, addiction and thereby they deviate from normal behavior.

The magnitude of the use of diverse platforms of social media has turned out to be a cause for apprehension in latest times, studies from the field of psychology, psychiatry is essential to tackle the complications due to this issue. The extensive use of social networking in India has been on the ascend especially in the midst of the adolescents; since they are the future citizens, it is vital to protect their mental health and hence this study is chosen. The study is entitled as "INFLUENCE OF SOCIAL NETWORKING ON MENTAL HEALTH AMONG ADOLESCENTS".

1.4 RESEARCH GAP

Very limited research has been conducted to comprehend the influence of social networking on mental health. There are only very limited studies that focus on the extent and pattern of social networking and the influence of various socio-demographic variables on social networking and mental health. There appears to be a paucity of research undertaken in social networking in the general education sector, signifying a gap in which research can be undertaken that can offer novel insight and add together with information. Mixed methodology approach is rarely adopted by the researchers, can help comprehend the topic area in better depth and help enhance assurance in the results / outcome of the study, providing more evidence while offsetting probable shortcomings from using one research approach (Bryman, A., & Cramer, D. 2004).

Prior researches chiefly ponder on the various factors separately, focus was given to the selected aspects in particular and priority was given more to mental illness. It is hoped that this study will pile up the space in the literature, as the researcher could not come across detailed studies conducted in the nation investigating the effects of social networking among adolescents, based on the specified demographic variables. A key goal of the psychiatric epidemiological research is to identify changeable factors interrelated to adolescent mental health. With this aim, the present study underpinned to explore the adolescent's social networking and mental health outcome. Various reasons for social networking, the impacts related to social networking, relation between impacts and addiction, mental health will provide a clear picture of the issue.

1.5 RESEARCH QUESTIONS

Research question plays a vital role in guiding a researcher in his / her work. The purpose and focus of the study, clarity of the research and its outcome is analysed through the research question. In thesis, there will be multiple questions which are connected well and focus on the major theme. The research questions identified in this study were the following:

1. How the adolescents will differ in socio demographic profile with respect to the engagement in social networking?
2. How the adolescents will differ in socio demographic profile with respect to their mental health?
3. What are the reasons for engaging in social networking?
4. How the impact of social networking does leads to addiction?
5. Whether social networking addiction influence mental health?

1.6 THEORETICAL SOURCES OF THE STUDY

1.6.1 Previous Theories Used in Social Networking and Mental Health

The current study is envisioned to address the gap by exploring the social networking and related issues through self-determination and cognitive behavioral model. There are many theories which talk about motivation, drive, need and the after effect of need satisfaction; addictive behaviors. But the lacunae is that no single theory provides the exact cause and effect; relation behind social networking and mental health.

1.6.2 Self Determination Theory

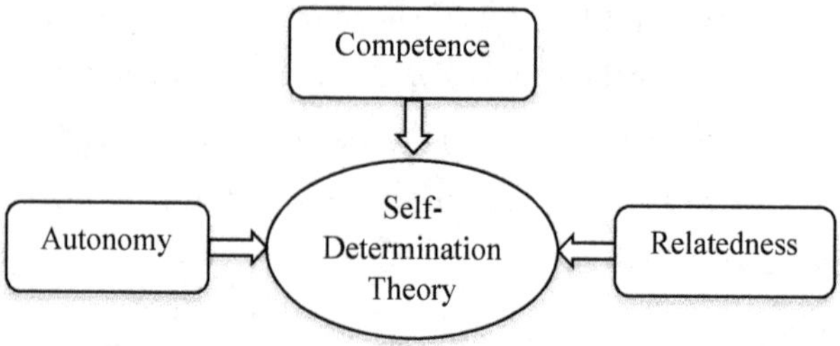

Figure 1.1 Self Determination Theory (Ryan and Deci, 2006)

The fundamental psychological needs of autonomy, competence, and relatedness; the essential part in self-determined motivation, well-being, and development is centered in this theory. These needs are said to be universal, innate and psychological, arise from the underlying motivations of an individual. Autonomy enhances need satisfaction and mental wellbeing (Deci, E. L., et al 2006). Social networking is an integral part of adolescent's lives and they can't imagine a life without being connected. This is an "always on' lifestyle", the youngsters hook up in social networking in order to connect (Boyd, D. 2007). Social networking enriches the feeling of closeness / relatedness / connectedness. It is a way of being and relating (Kuss, D. J., & Griffiths, M. D. 2017). Virtual space is created by the adolescent social networking users and this serve the need to belong (Boyd, D. 2014).

This enhances autonomy as per Nadkarni, A., & Hofmann, S. G. (2012). Competence is the sense of mastery, arises out of curiosity and autonomy refers to freedom, contentment from choosing one's own independent views. Social networking is easily available and accessible. Hence it can satisfy ones needs virtually in a fast manner. Weinstein, N., et al (2017) applied self-determination theory on 5,777 adults in America to examine the effect of motivation and its related factors on internet gaming disorder. The prospective study found that need satisfaction influenced health positively; prevents internet gaming disorder.

Kircaburun, K., et al (2019) scanned the problems associated with social networking in 760 college students. Convenience sampling method was adopted and standardized tools were used. The results revealed issues related to social networking-cyber bullying was more among high school boys. Belongingness is directly associated with cyber bullying and connectedness is indirectly associated with problematic social networking.

Berezan, O., et al (2020) explored the factors that influence social networking; the study took self-determination theory viewpoint. Through random sampling technique the researchers selected 323 US citizens. The study proved that people who are lonely will get into social networking for interaction and belongingness, the two essential psychological needs for an individual. The clarification of self-determination theory remains blurred. There are unanswered interrogations. What are the other needs to be satisfied? What are the antecedents that lead one to need satisfaction? Whether any mediators in need satisfaction? What is the after effect?

Through the extensive review, the researcher found other factors which contribute to the wide influence of social networking and social networking addiction. The nature of social networking, multiple factors associated with social networking and the various purposes of social networking such as entertainment, interaction, information and online shopping can satisfy the person. Accessibility; availability and anonymity act as the reinforcing stimulus.

1.6.3 Cognitive Behavioral Theory

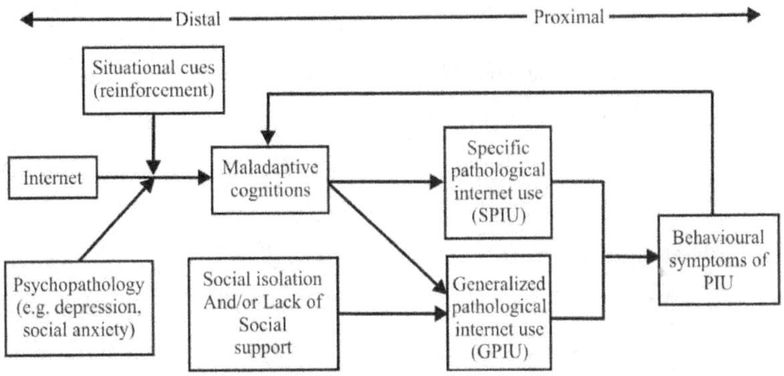

Figure 1.2 Cognitive Behavioral Model (Davis 2001)

If the teenager is not satisfied in life; he / she has unmet needs, features of mental illness can arise at any point in the transition period. Behavioral and mental issues can arise because of the increased social networking or else the signs and symptoms can aggravate if, the person is not mentally healthy (Ryan, R. M., & Deci, E. L. 2000; Chak, K., & Leung, L. 2004; Ebeling-Witte, S., et al 2007).

In Davis's model, the stressor which may boost the pathological use of internet is social networking. As per the cognitive behavioral model, anxiety and depression act as catalyst in social networking. The cognitive behavioral model portrays only the negative side of social networking.

Wong, T. Y., et al (2015) used need theory and cognitive behavioral model approach; formulated and proved a model: need fulfilment leads to knotty internet use with psychosocial agony as mediators. The items in need satisfaction were relatedness, competence and autonomy. The mediating factors in psychosocial distress were anxiety and depression. The features of addiction (preference, tolerance, mood changes, dependence and problems) were explored in problematic internet use.

1.6.4 Social Stimulation Hypothesis, Social Displacement Hypothesis

Social networking can influence social relationship and ultimately distress the mental health. Social stimulation hypothesis was proposed by McKenna et al (2000) and Social displacement hypothesis was proposed by Kraut et al (1998).

Social stimulation hypothesis argues that social networking contributes positively to social relationships, mental health. The researchers Morgan, C., & Cotten, S. R. (2003); Bessière, K., et al (2008) theorised that adolescents like forming relations, become close with others through social networking and can have good mental health. Social displacement hypothesis states that social media affects negatively on teenage social relationships, mental health. People interact with others through social networking and it can create positive and negative emotions. From this theory it is lucid that social networking can have positive as well as negative impact on mental health.

Valkenburg, P. M., & Peter, J. (2013) focussed on the differential susceptibility to media effects model (DSMM). They emphasise that media can cause problems both physical and mental, is motivated by the type of device used, personal factors (socioeconomic factors, personality).Thus the connection between social networking and mental health depend on other factors that have not yet been investigated.

The proposed theoretical model explains the antecedents that can lead to social networking. These antecedents contribute to the need satisfaction. That is the nature and factors associated with social networking; pattern and purpose of social networking influences the social networking of an adolescent. The nature of social networking can act as a reinforce, which include low cost, easy access, privacy, curiosity, acceptance, freedom, satisfying need, feeling of internet as a part of life / everything is available in it etc. The poor mental health / mental illness corroborate the connection between need satisfaction and social networking addiction.

In this context mental health is assessed through Warwick-Edinburgh tool. The final outcome of social networking is that it affects the mental health. The constructive and unconstructive side of social networking is focussed in this study. In order to test this model, the researcher selected 840 middle adolescents; as the review says "mental illness is more in the period of identity change" (Morahan-Martin, J., & Schumacher, P. 2000; Widyanto, L., & Griffiths, M. 2006; Yen, C. F., et al 2009).

1.7 CONCEPTUAL FRAMEWORK

In current years, the upsurge of social networking users has directed to the development of multidisciplinary research focussing on the bright and dark side linked with it. The intention is to explore the hidden reasons associated with social networking, social networking addiction and the various social networking impacts on mental health. The framework is related to social networking and mental health; highlights reasons for social networking, social networking impacts, social networking addiction and mental health. In the proposed conceptual framework, social networking is the independent variable whereas mental health is measured as dependent variable.

The figure shows unidirectional relationship of social networking impacts-social networking addiction, social networking addiction-mental health.

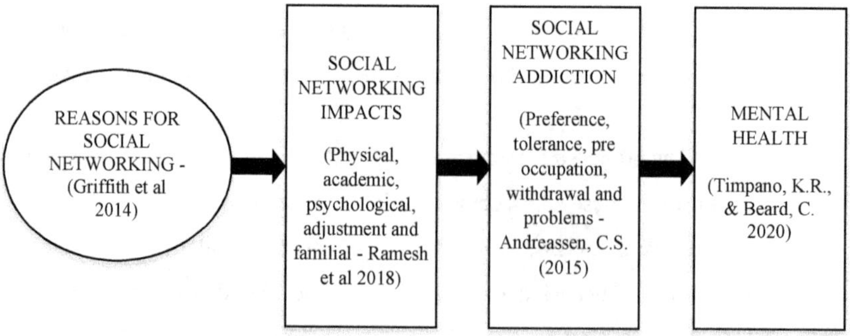

Figure 1.3 Conceptual Framework

1.8 OBJECTIVES

The present study was framed with the following objectives.

- Objective 1: To assess the difference in socio demographic profile on the basis of social networking addiction and mental health.
- Objective 2: To identify the reasons for engaging in social networking.
- Objective 3: To explore the relationship between reasons and impacts of social networking on addiction and mental health.
- Objective 4: To assess the influence of social networking impacts on mental health.
- Objective 5: To analyse the most influential impact of social networking on mental health.
- Objective 6: To develop a model on influence of social networking on mental health
- Objective 7: To explore the influence of social networking on mental health through qualitative analysis.

1.9 HYPOTHESIS OF THE STUDY

- HI: There is significant difference in socio demographic variables with respect to social networking addiction and mental health.
- H2: There is significant relationship between reasons and impacts of social networking with social networking addiction, mental health.
- H3: There is significant influence of social networking impact on social networking addiction.
- H4: There is significant influence of social networking impact on mental health.

1.10 SCOPE OF THE STUDY

The **Scope** of the study can be condensed as follows.

1. The present study investigated the influence of social networking on mental health of middle adolescents. The study analyzes the current mental health position of the adolescent students in relation to social networking behavior, identifies the constraints and hurdles to overcome to keep up the adolescent's mental health.
2. The baseline implications of the study provide insight into the mental health issues among adolescents and provide pointers towards policy development and suggest strategies to meet the challenges in the mental health issues of adolescent learners.
3. The study pinpoints the present status of social networking behavior and the mental health of middle adolescents; this understanding will assist to outline the scope of viable changes to be made in general education and health department's policy and programs.
4. The rigorous examination of adolescent's social networking behavior and its influence on their mental health will have the potential to inform the

design of educational and health interventions, development of preventive programs and define strategy options to reduce the negative impacts among adolescents.

1.11 OPERATIONAL DEFINITION OF KEY TERMS

1.11.1 Influence

Influence is the control or capability of bringing an effect on an individual in tortuous or insubstantial ways (Dictionary, M. W. 2002). In the present study, the term *influence* is used in the same sense, that is, *the* ability to cause desirable and measurable actions and outcomes on the mental health of middle adolescent social networking users.

1.11.2 Social Networking

Social networking is the employ of fanatical websites and its applications to relate with others, or to locate citizens with like interests to one's own (Dictionary, O. E. 1989). In the present study, the term *social networking* is used in the same way that is, the method of constructing, fostering virtual groups and associations online between middle adolescents.

1.11.3 Mental Health

Mental Health is a state of comfort in which the person realizes his or her own abilities, can handle with the usual stress of life, can work effectively, productively, and is able to make a contribution to his or her community (World Health Organization). In the present study, the term *Mental Health* is used in the same sense. The study focuses on the mental health of middle adolescent social networking users.

1.11.4 Adolescent

Adolescence is an intermediary stage of growth and development between childhood and adulthood. The age group of adolescent is between 10-19 (World

Health Organization, 2006). In the present study, an adolescent means a student aged 15 to 17 years (middle adolescents) only.

1.12 CHAPTERISATION

The research report consists of five chapters.

Chapter One contains the introduction of the study, need for the study, statement of the problem, research gap identified, research questions, objectives, hypothesis, theoretical back ground, conceptual model developed, scope of the research and operational definition of the main terms in the study. From this chapter one will get a clear idea about the relevance of the study in the present period.

Chapter Two deals with the review of related studies. Extensive literature review was done on reasons for social networking, reasons for social networking habit, purpose of engaging in social networking, social networking impacts, social networking addiction and its influence on mental health. Review was also done on the various social networking sites, the mediators of social networking and the prevalence of the problem to get a clear picture about the recent social networking behavior of the adolescents.

Chapter Three explains the research methodology in detail. The research design, various phases of the study, overview of the research process, sampling framework including the sampling technique, sample size and its calculation, scale development after pilot study, scales used in the study and the statistical tools used was explained clearly in this chapter. The importance of sequential explanatory mixed method is evident in this chapter.

Chapter Four is devoted to analysis of the data. Descriptive and inferential statistics is used in this study. This chapter contains Frequency analysis, Mean analysis, Anova, T test, Correlation analysis, Multiple regression, Confirmatory factor analysis, Structural equation modelling and thematic analysis. The statistical tools used were SPSS-20, AMOS-22 and NVIVO-12.

Chapter Five gives the discussion of findings, summary, conclusions, implications, recommendations and suggestions for further research. The findings of the study is interpreted and discussed well with the previous research findings. Recommendations need to be implemented in order to prevent mental illness and to promote mental health. Bibliography and appendices are given at the last after the final chapter.

CHAPTER 2

REVIEW OF LITERATURE

2.1 INTRODUCTION

Review of literature is of considerable importance to the researcher because, through the recognition and scrutiny of related past studies that contain details pertinent to the present study, it gives awareness to the researcher regarding the significance of the problem. In the initial stage of research, the literature helps the researcher to familiarize with the problem area. The basic outcome of the review of literature becomes the "frame of reference" for research. Review of literature help the researcher to comprehend the issue, formulate working hypothesis and keep away from pointless duplication. The present chapter provides an apparent review based on social networking and mental health; categorised under various headings such as reasons for preferring social networking, reasons for social networking addiction, its pattern and purpose, beneficial and harmful impacts of social networking, social networking and mental health.

One of the latest study on internet addiction in Rajasthan, India by **Jain, A., et al (2020)** evaluated the prevalence, pattern of internet addiction and the occurrence of mental health issues due to internet addiction among 954 adolescent students. Addiction, depression and insomnia was assessed through standardized questionnaires. The results highlighted that 43.19% students were increasingly using internet and 15.51% were addicted to internet. 19.81% were over users / addicted and used internet for more than 2 hours / day. Addiction was more among boys. Internet usage time was positively correlated with addiction in internet. Poor sleep and depression was noted among addicts.

2.2 SOCIAL NETWORKING

This section deals with the various factors leading to social networking, the pattern of social networking and the purpose of social networking that directly / indirectly influence social networking.

2.2.1 Reasons for Social Networking

Huffstutler, S., et al (2002) pointed out that through social networking, any relevant matter pertaining to education / work can be accessed easily and this is the reason for increased social networking. **Caplan, S. E. (2003)** conducted a study among 386 individuals with the help of Generalized Problematic Internet Use Scale (GPIUS). Depression and loneliness was noted to be noteworthy predictors of inclination for online social interaction. Increased social networking was more among people with feeling of loneliness, depression. The study emphasised that in order to change the mood, people engage in social networking and can land up with destructive effects.

Caplan, S. E. (2005) discovered mental health / mental wellbeing, as the origin and the end product of internet use". **Ito, M., & Okabe, D. (2005)** found that feeling of loneliness is relieved through social networking. **Gemmill, E. L., & Peterson, M. (2006)** ensured that social networking has an unavoidable part in youngster's life and hence they engage in it. Thus accommodation acts as a factor in social networking. **Goodman, J. (2007)** tested the involvement of college students in technology, social networking. He pointed out - "Social Networking Sites are not a fraction of student's lives, in reality they are their lives". "Adolescents are not only the early adopters of the novel technologies, but they are moreover among the most polished users as well".

Zywica, J., & Danowski, J. (2008) concluded from the study that those who are panic in face-to-face communication and fear on in person interaction feel less lonely, when they engage in social networking and hence use it excessively. **Park, S. K., et al (2008)** studied the prevalence of social networking addiction and its factors among 903 middle adolescents, Korea. 10.7% users were at risk for addiction, found that family bonding and effective parenting are the factors that prevent addiction in teenagers. **Yen, C. F., et al (2009)** found association of hostility and depression with internet addiction. **Johnson, L., et al (2009)** mentioned that people use social networking regularly because of the experiences that they get and due to on-going attraction. **Bernardi, S., & Pallanti, S. (2009)** assessed nine girl students, measured the comorbidities. Symptoms were screened carefully. The study identified that six male students were affected with internet addiction, had features of anxiety and personality disorder.

Pujazon-Zazik, M., & Park, M. J. (2010) reviewed studies on use of online media, gender differences, parental monitoring of adolescents engaged in social media and health outcomes due to the social networking. The reviewer concluded that risk taking behavior can be avoided through monitoring by parents; otherwise it can land up with online sex / addiction to sex videos / cyber bullying and can give individual details to sexual predators. Thus lack of parental monitoring is a factor in social networking. **Jairak, R., et al (2010)** explored the factors that influence social networking. The researchers identified that the factor behind social networking is the purpose for which people engage in social networking. **Valtysson, B. (2010)** reported that, social networking is flexible and hence youngster prefers it.

Das, B., & Sahoo, J. S. (2011) found that virtual communication / interaction is fostered through social networking, as people can express the opinion and there by freedom is delivered in social networking. Thus freedom promotes adolescents to engage in social networking. **Griffiths, M. D., et al (2014), Ryan, T., & Xenos, S. (2011)** mentioned, social networking allows escapism from unpleasant situations and negative feelings. **Ahn, J. (2011)** studied the result of social networking on student's development; teenage students were enchanted by social networking. Privacy is ensured in social networking / chat rooms and hence adolescent feel more comfortable in social networking. Security, time spend, academic achievement, physical and mental health concern and are the worries noted among parents. **Lin, K. Y., & Lu, H. P. (2011)** noted enjoyment as the major reason behind social networking among students. **Parveen, N. (2011)** stated that in order to keep updated about the news and knowledge, people engage in social networking, Facebook.

Nadkarni, A., & Hofmann, S. G. (2012) identified that in order to connect with others, people engage in social networking. People need sense of belongingness, a need of self-presentation and hence they engage in social networking. **Toma, C. L., & Hancock, J. T. (2013)** found out that Facebook helps to satisfy people, hence engage in social networking. **Rosen, L. D., et al (2013)** stated that people engage in social networking to have more friends, increased number of online friends is associated with features of depression, mania and personality disorder. **Calisir, F., et al (2013)** identified the factors influencing social networking through a survey among 155 students. Ease of use, fun and influence of others are the factors associated with social networking.

Gómez Salgado, P., et al (2014) interviewed 2339 secondary school students in Galicia, for problematic internet use. The data was collected with 20 students in one group at a time and revealed their internet habits, magnitude of the problem. 60.4% of teenagers agreed that they accessed internet daily / almost every day. 26.8% accessed internet once or twice a week. 45.8% used internet 1-2 hours a day, 10.5% accessed internet for more than 3 hours daily. 56.8% connected internet between 16.00-21.00, 39.2% connected between 21.00-12.00 and 6% connected from midnight. 36.2% of the youngsters stated that they are not on internet all the time they would like. 55% accessed internet in their own room, and 15.8% were using their mobile phones for surfing. 54% responded lack of parental control, in using internet. 77.9% argued rarely / never with their parents regarding internet use, 6.3% had problems frequently and 14.6% had problems in between. 64.3% used internet to download music, movies and photos.

Wegmann, E., et al (2015) studied social networking addiction, occurrence of depression / anxiety among the 334 participants. The researchers found that youngsters engage in social networking in order to get rid of the negative feelings. **Riva, G., et al (2015)** stated that social networking meets all basic human needs and this is the reason observed among adolescent social networking users. The various needs include safety, security, association, love, belongingness and self-realization. **Krol, P. C., et al (2015)** has completed a study on – "The Role of Social Anxiety in Adolescents Social Media Use", to locate the outcome of social anxiety on social networking among 415 adolescents (15-18 years). The study showed that anxiety is a predictor of social networking addiction; study indicated a clear correlation between anxiety and social networking. Gender, education level and type of school were predictors of social networking.

Sharma, I., & Sharma, N. (2016) directed a study regarding the use of social networking among 400 adolescents (200 boys and girls) aged 16-18years, Jammu. Multistage sampling technique was used. The adolescents mainly engage in social networking through mobile and they were having profile in social networking sites. The preferred site was Facebook. They engage in social networking for chatting, status updating and sharing photos. The participants started account in social networking sites before the age of 18 years and the parents never stopped from doing so. **Pradeep, P., & Sriram, S. (2016)** assessed the usage of social networking among 121 youngsters of age 13-18 years in the metropolitan city, Mumbai, India. The results showed increased accessibility to the internet and the origin of smart phones, its availability resulted in increased social networking. The factors that prevent youngsters from social networking include parental supervision and monitoring.

Kristianto, B. (2017) assessed the factors related to social networking use among 460 primary school students, Indonesia. The factors reported include influence of friends / parents, easy access of social networking. **Raj, M., et al (2018)** administered questionnaire in secret on 388 students to verify the pattern of social networking on educational performance among the school students of Siliguri, West Bengal, India. They found that 87.1% students connect in social networking, engage in an augmented amount of time in it. 70.7% were addicted to social networking, addiction was more among 17 years and above. The sites visited were WhatsApp 277 (82%), followed by Facebook 254 (75.1%) and Instagram -114 users (33.7%). Students accessed social networking through smart phones 256 (75.7%) and computers at home 207 (61.5%). The regularity of inspection speckled in excess, five times a day 102 (30.2%). 110 students (32.5%) alleged that social networking ruined the school performance.

Sowndarya, T. A., & Pattar, M. (2018) focussed on the prevalence of addiction to internet and the related factors in school students, Mangalore, India. 83.3% addiction was among the urban school students; whereas in rural school students it was 71%. The risk factors were gender-boys, owning smart phone, unceasing obtainability of internet (availability), pornography, the time they engage online and the peer influence. **Guraya, S. Y., et al (2018)** checked the extent and nature of social networking among 1181 adults, Kuwait and Saudi. 52% used social networking sites for academic purpose, 38% shared lectures through it. **Kırcaburun, K., & Griffiths, M. D. (2019)** conducted a self-reported study to look at the connection between the murky behavior with social networking among 772 University students in Nottingham, United Kingdom. The result indicated positive association with respect to male gender and increased involvement in social networking.

Abbas, J., et al (2019) selected 831students from Pakistan for evaluating the engagement in social networking. Social gratification theory is applied in this study. People engage in social networking to reduce stress, to maintain contact, to increase confidence and to increase knowledge level. The negative impacts of social networking include cyber bullying, laziness, time wasting, anxiety and depression. Thus the researchers concluded that adolescents benefit less from social networking when compared to the harmful risks due to this behavior. **Kushlev, K., & Leitao, M.R. (2020)** supervised the smart phone usage and studied the effect of mobile on well-being. The results projected that increased smart phone use for social networking can cause decreased well-being. **Aparicio-Martínez, P., et al (2020)** assessed the factors influencing social networking through a cross-sectional study among 278 adolescents studying in college. The results revealed that social networking is related to factors such as gender, social, psychological and biological factors.

2.2.2 Reasons for Social Networking Addiction

Morahan-Martin, J., & Schumacher, P. (2000) lead an assessment of 277 college students (150 boys and 127 girls) to measure the occurrence and correlates of online issues. The study used 13 questionnaires related to academic, occupational, social problems and addiction. Study showed that students with heavy use "pathological users" (8.1%), mild use - "limited symptoms" (64.7%) and with no symptoms - "NO symptoms" (27.2%). Increased utilisation of social networking especially for online sex, games was more observed in pathological users and it was more in boys. The researchers emphasized that when one start engaging in social networking, they develop compulsion towards it, feel like using every time and can have impacts. **Ceyhan, E. (2007)** studied the relationship between heavy internet use and gender among the 437 college students. The study found that the factors such as gender, social networking during night time, symptoms of mental illness, using it for entertainment, predicted the problematic use.

Mythily, S., et al (2008) surveyed 2735 youngsters with respect to their social networking using a 69 - item questionnaire. Demographic profile, academic presentation, social support, overall wellbeing and purpose of social networking were explored. The youngsters who fritter more than 5 hours per day in internet were classified as heavy users; 17.1% respondents were heavy users. 49.3% were boys and 50.6% were girls. 25% were not accessing internet daily. The factors that contribute to the increase in social networking were sad mood, poor academic performance and lack of rules at home. **Ni, X., et al (2009)** studied 3557 college students in China regarding their social networking behavior. The research concluded that 6.44% had addiction and depression / anxiety was more noted among the addicts. The factors associated with addiction include age of first exposure to social networking, single-parent and place of residence-urban.

Yao, B., et al (2013) has done a case control cohort study to identify the mental health deviations due to heavy internet use among 977 students in a university; China. The study discovered various causal factors such as anxiety, depression-predictors of online addiction. **Aksoy, L., et al (2013)** found out the reasons behind social networking addiction within the twenty five university students, in Turkey through a qualitative study. The addiction was due to deficient in friends, inevitability of social media, sentiment of accomplishment and fear of missing out. **Sasmaz, T., et al (2013)** has examined the risk factors and prevalence rate of social networking addiction in 1156 students attending high school in Mersin Province. Addiction was more prevalent in the current samples. Results emphasized that 79% own computer, 9.3% females and 20.4% males were addicted. Independent relationship was observed between gender, year of study, hobby, duration of social networking, depression and addiction.

Li, C., et al (2014) performed a study regarding the influence of behavior of parents and self-control on social networking addiction among 966 adolescents in middle school, China. The findings revealed that there were 51 students with high risk for addiction; males were addicted more than females. Students with internet addiction showed lesser mean score for positive support from parents. **Li, W., et al (2014)** analyzed the familial factors leading to social networking addiction among youngsters, China. Youngsters with problematic internet use / internet addiction reported family disorganization, dissatisfaction, conflict between parents / between parent and child. Addiction was noted more among adults with divorced parents and single parent.

Yao, M. Z., et al (2014) identified the factors that have an influence on internet addiction. The survey was done among 2,905 students in a university, China. The findings showed that rejection of parents was positively correlated with addiction. Factors that supplement addiction include personality, behavior of parents and self-esteem. An increased risk for internet addiction was also noted among students with overprotected fathers. **Andreassen, C. S. (2015)** explored the association between various addiction such as Facebook, online games, internet, mobile, shopping and personality among 218 students from a university. The study showed positive association between the seven subtypes of addiction. Neuroticism; emotional instability, lack of control, poor ability to manage stress, maladjustment was positively associated with addiction on internet. Extroversion; positive emotion was positively associated with addiction towards Facebook, online shopping and mobile.

Kirik, A., et al (2015) focused on social networking among 271, 13 – 19 years old students in Turkey. The researchers observed the fact that social networking addiction is low in 14 year old adolescents, as the age progresses the addiction increases till 17 years and it reduces after that. Irrespective of the age, people get attracted towards social networking. Addictive nature increases as the time spend in social networking increases. The factors-age, time spend in social networking; number of visits to social networking is associated with addiction to social networking. **Braun, B., et al (2016)** conducted a research to identify the role of religion in gaming, whether engagement in prayer, spiritual life affect gaming behavior.5990 men participated in the cohort study. From the investigation it was clear that, people practicing Christianity has involved in less frequent gaming-online and had less game addiction when compared to people without religious denomination. Thus the study concluded that religious belief was related to less gaming behavior.

Gill, K. J., et al (2016) conducted a survey on gaming, addiction and psychological health among people of Quebec Cree community. Sample size was 506. Standardized tool on depression, addiction was used. The survey identified that 69.2% engaged in gambling / games, moderate / high risk gamblers were 20.6% and severe problematic ones were 3.2%. Females played games more often than males. Anxiety, depression and stressful life events were the risk factors for problematic gambling. **Sharma, M. K., et al (2017)** has done a survey on internet addiction among 2755 personalities (1392 men and 1363 women), Bangalore, India. The findings showed internet addiction among 1.3%, excessive mobile phone use among 4.1%. Clients from single families were addicted more, less addiction is found in nuclear and joint families.

Biolcati, R., et al (2018) examined the boredom proneness among 478 adolescents in Italy. Usage of technology was more among teenagers with boredom feeling, absence of hobbies / extracurricular activities. The study concluded that in order to avoid boredom, adults engage in social networking. **Su, B., et al (2018)** conducted study among 1490 adolescents and found that excessive social networking can be prevented through good parental monitoring and good father - child relationship. **Gorman, T. E., et al (2018)** mentioned that online games are one of the most accepted entertainments in social networking. Gaming is considered as a common form of entertainment among females than male adults; 90% of the youngsters engage in it and they are more prone for excessive social networking. Few people who play video games had negative impacts and some had features of addiction. **Kim, Y. J., et al (2018)** explored the factors that influence increased social networking among 653 school students, Korea. Addiction, mood, temperament, and social interactions were assessed. Males spend more time in social networking for gaming and this is the major factor behind social networking addiction.

Kırcaburun, K., & Griffiths, M. D. (2019) explored the role of social networking in real life. 333 users of Instagram (14-23years) participated in this study. The study showed that in order to escape from reality, real life situations, adolescents engage in social networking. Escapism act as a mediator in problematic internet use. **Kircaburun, K., et al (2019)** tried to find out the relation between problematic social networking and cyber bullying. Two sets of samples were taken - 804 and 760 respectively. The study revealed strong association between problematic social networking and cyber bullying. **Yurdagül, C., et al (2019)** examined the psychological impacts of problematic social networking among 491 adolescents between 14-19 years. The study found association between problematic social networking and depression, anxiety, loneliness. **Kircaburun, K., et al (2019)** assessed the association between addiction in online games and psychological problems. A comprehensive survey was done among 242 participants. The study found features of depression as a key risk factor in increased / problematic online gaming.

Mamun, M. A., et al (2019) explored the prevalence and risk factors in social networking addiction through a cross-sectional study among 284 students, Bangladesh. The sampling technique was convenience sampling. The findings revealed that 3.9% of the participants were using internet in an excessive amount, those who engage in social networking for over 5 hours per day and poor mental health are more prone for addiction. **Mamun, M. A., et al (2020)** examined the internet use associated issues through a cross-sectional study among 605 students, Bangladesh. The risk factors identified were loneliness, stress, online chatting, sleep problems and using internet not for educational purpose. **Hussain, Z., et al (2020)** identified the social networking and related disorders in 466 adolescents (early and middle adolescents, 10-17 years) from higher secondary school.99.4% agreed that their preferred social networking site is Whatsapp and majority of the participants were active in one social networking site. The study proved that belongingness is an essential need in adolescence period and in order to satisfy this need, they engage in social networking. Thus need to belong is a factor that lead teens to problematic social networking.

2.2.3 Pattern of Social Networking

Anderson, C. A., & Bushman, B. J. (2001) conducted one of the chief studies in social networking among 1300 college students from eight universities. The study noted, the average time spent daily in online by the students was 99 minutes. **Lin, S. S., & Tsai, C. C. (2002)** analysed the internet use of 753 high school students, Taiwan. Dependence to internet was found among those who spend more time online. The chance of dependence is more if the adolescent had early exposure in social networking. **Nalwa, K., & Anand, A. P. (2003)** in their study revealed that 17% of the internet dependents spent 1-30 minutes daily on online activities, 50% took 1-2 hours daily, 28% 2-4 hours and 5.5 % spent extra than overall. The researchers noted that addicted users have poor academic performance. **Yang, S. C., & Tung, C. J. (2007)** has done a study among 1708 adolescents, Taiwanese high school students. The examiners found addiction in 236 teens and they used to spend double amount of time in social networking than the non addicts. The addiction towards internet has negatively influenced the student's academics, relationship and daily routines. **Tsitsika, A., et al (2009)** assessed 897 teenagers from Greece regarding the internet usage. The assessment identified that one of the predictors of use was accessing internet via one's own home, as this ensures privacy. Excessive social networking was seen among those who play online games.

Song, X. Q., et al (2010) has done a research on the epidemiological characteristics, factors of addiction in internet, among 1219 students in Wuhan city. The results revealed that the place for surfing act as a factor for addiction. **Bringula, R., et al (2012)** identified the pattern of social networking, measured in terms of hours spent and time of social networking. The sample size was 545, the research design adopted was exploratory-descriptive design and the setting was Manila. Foremost social networking usage was among male adolescents, more than half of the participants owned computer at home, but they were visitors of internet café also. **Kochhar, S., et al (2013)** discovered that half of the engineering students pointed out that they preferred to use internet at home. **Yadav, P., et al (2013)** has done a study among 11th and 12th students in India, found that the addicted students spend a mean of 2.5 hours (S.D = 2.3) per day online. The researchers mentioned that out of the 522 questionnaires filled by the students, all the students were accessing internet at home. 3.2% of the respondents accessed internet from both home and cyber cafe.

Goel, D., et al (2013) identified that most of the internet addicts used internet in the dusk and evening; whereas non addicts used in the sunrise and early afternoon. **Salehan, M., & Negahban, A. (2013)** checked the usage of mobile phone in youngsters. The use of mobile application depends on the amount of social networking. **Kumar, A., & Kumar, R. (2013)** assessed the influence of social networking sites in the middle of 150 students in Punjab, India. The main purpose of social networking was for entertainment -92.66%, followed by sharing videos / pictures, messaging and for information gain. 46.67% had 10-49 friends, 33.33% had 50-100 friends in social networking sites. Facebook was the most preferred site among the youngsters. 73.33% used mobile for accessing social networking. Among the respondents, 53.33% faced lack of time, 6.67% felt social networking as not secure, 5.33% felt lack of privacy, 3.33% felt it was not user friendly and 26.67% identified poor connectivity. 4.67% had lack of technical understanding and 47.33% experienced easiness in social networking. 20% students were highly satisfied with social networking; whereas 7.33% were not satisfied with it. 47.33% agreed that social networking is reliable; while 22.67% found it as not reliable.

Sultan, A. J. (2014) studied addiction, stated from the findings of his study that the application of text messaging is addicted to mobile services. **Griffiths, M. D., et al (2014)** the use of social networking sites has quickly become ubiquitous and in particular among adolescents and young adults. Social networking is the chosen virtual activity of teenagers. **De Cock, R., et al (2014)** evaluated 1000 Belgian adults regarding their internet use, usage of social networking sites. The study checked the period disbursed on internet / social networking sites, stage of development, gender, education, income, occupation, holiday time activities. The study revealed that gender and age explained a major part of the increased usage. **Shabir, G., et al (2014)** has done a research on social networking impacts in 300 teenagers. The participants were influenced by social networking and the most used site was Facebook. 46 percent of the teenagers connect social networking from the institution they study. **Bruno, A., et al (2014)** has done an appraisal on the occurrence of internet addiction among Italian high school students. Variables include age, gender, place of residence and type of internet activity. From the assessment they found that there was no effect of the place of residence on internet addiction.

Sharma, S. K., et al (2016) monitored the pattern, engagement in social networking sites among 550 adolescent undergraduate students, Dehradun, India. In case of males, face book (96.58%) was the most preferred site followed by Whatsapp (83.65%); whereas in case of females Whatsapp (71.22%) was the preferred site followed by Facebook (67.15%). 98.10% males and 93.73% females accessed social networking from mobile phones. 94.68% students engage in social networking for fun. Other purposes include education and to contact friends. **Demetrovics, Z., et al (2016)** studied the internet use related problems among adolescents. The study revealed that 77.7% engaged in social networking, 68.8% of the participants used internet during leisure hours. 68.4% used social networking for chatting, 57.8% for entertainment, 45.5% for gaining information, 23.8% for online gaming and 8.0% for sending emails. Those who squander over 6 hours per day in internet are prone for problematic behavior; they showed decreased academic performance, reduced confidence and increased depressive features. **Mmin, M. (2017)** has done a study related to online addiction among 300 college students, Haryana. The study showed that 59.66% students accessed internet through computer, 72% owned smart phone. The purpose of social networking among 43.33% was to gain knowledge. 59% of students faced problems due to intermittent usage.

Bharati, V. K., & Singh, M. P. (2018) assessed the social networking through a descriptive survey among 200 students, Varanasi, India. The study found Whatsapp and Facebook as the most preferred sites by the students and the purpose of engaging in social networking was for education and interaction. **Saini, N., et al (2020)** implemented a cross sectional study to appraise the influence of social networking among 220 youngsters of age 18-21 years, Chandigarh, India. The main aim of using internet by the participants was for social networking (57%). 22% engage in social networking for chatting, 67% to connect with the friends and 48% in order to gain information. 97% responded that the preferred social networking site was Facebook. The type of device used by 56% was mobile phone; the place of accessing social networking by 35% was from home. 58% visited social networking site once a day. 3% engaged in social networking during school hours. The adolescents recognised waste of time (31%) and hacking (20%) in social networking. Stress was perfectly handled by the daily users of social networking.

2.2.4 Purpose of Social Networking

Livingstone, S. (1998) stated that the purpose of social networking by students is to interact with family members. **Munt, S. R., et al (2002)** mentioned that people connect with others through social networking. **Lampe, C. A., et al (2007)** surveyed 286 adolescents, tried to observe the purpose of social networking. The students used social networking to enhance the old relations and to get in touch with friends. The usage boosted the self-esteem, life satisfaction and ultimately the mental wellbeing. **Vitak, J. (2008)** emphasised that the major reason of social networking is to contact strangers and to establish relation with them through chatting / messaging.

Tahiroglu, A. Y., et al (2008) identified various habits of internet use among the 3975 adolescents, Turkey. They found that 7.6% of the adolescents engage in social networking for more than 12 hours per week. The reasons for social networking was playing online games; which was more seen in males and gaining information; which was more noted in girls. **Coyle, C. L., & Vaughn, H. (2008)** conducted a survey among 68 youngsters regarding the social networking habit. The findings of the open-ended questions displayed that teens keep in touch with friends (41%), socialize through social networking and the frequency of social networking visit was three times per day. **Subrahmanyam, K., et al (2008)** explored the social networking among teenagers. Youngsters read others profile / comment / post photos in social networking, engage in social networking mainly to connect with others.

Brandtzæg, P. B., & Heim, J. (2009) identified various reasons that motivate a person for social networking among 5233 adults. 31% engage in social networking to form new relations because of the loneliness / searching new friends, 21% to chat with friends, 14% to socialize in spare time, 3% to share videos / photos / pictures, 2% to have fun, 1.5% to surf and 10% to gain knowledge. 3% of the participants responded that they engage in social networking out of curiosity. Thus the researchers concluded that the purpose of social networking is based on the motivations / needs suggested in User Gratification Theory; information, entertainment, interaction and identity. **Tyson, J. (2009)** observed the social networking among 100 collegiate students, Carolina. The study findings suggested that 69% used to send messages, 16% like to post photos / play online games, 12% students like to surf and 3% were not having any purpose.

Korkeila, J., et al (2010) has distributed online questionnaires to 1825 students, with an aim to rule out the negatives hidden in the internet use. Negative correlation was found with addiction and social support. The main purpose of social networking was for fun, gaming and chatting. **Kuppuswamy, S., & Narayan, P. S. (2010)** discovered that teens are attracted towards social networking, mainly to open Whatsapp and Facebook. It helps in connecting with loved ones, but it affects academics negatively by distracting students from learning. **Mohamed, H. K., &**

Sumitha, E. (2011) observed the students of Calicut University, Kerala and found them sending messages, meeting new friends through social networking. **Khan, S. (2012)** performed a detailed study on the purpose of social networking. The sample size was 168. The respondents of the present study engage in social networking for fun, knowledge gain, time pass and for interaction. People start engaging in social networking due to peer influence.

Aillerie, K., & McNicol, S. (2018) studied the purpose of social networking by adolescent high school students. Even though students use social networking sites to gain academic information, it was not the most common purpose of social networking; they also use it for day to day information gaining. **Vela, K. (2018)** mentioned that academic libraries uses Facebook, twitter to connect with student users; helped in posting news, updates / announcements, doubts, there by enhanced collaboration and communication. **Kırcaburun, K., & Griffiths, M. D. (2019)** inspected the social networking sites and usage of 333 adolescents. The results project that only few showed problematic behavior. Adolescents who engage in social networking in order to escape from reality, displayed problematic social networking. **Kircaburun, K., et al (2020)** executed a study on excessive and problematic social networking among a convenience sample of 1008 students, Turkey. The most frequently used social networking site was WhatsApp (92%). The youngsters engage in social networking for maintaining relationships, meeting new individuals, to pass time, enjoyment and for gaining knowledge.

2.3 SOCIAL NETWORKING IMPACTS

The impacts of social networking in humane are very wide. If one has to know the overall impact, then the physical and mental health aspects have to be taken care of. This section deals with the positive, negative impacts and studies that display both the impacts of social networking.

2.3.1 Positive Impacts of Social Networking

Hartup, W. W., & Stevens, N. (1999) stated, social networking can prevent one from stress. **Subrahmanyam, K., et al (2000); Valentine, G., & Holloway, S. L. (2002)** emphasized, social networking is a means to fortify interpersonal relationships. **Reid, D., & Reid, F. (2004)** analysed the positive impact of technology in interpersonal communication and realised that it helps in developing interpersonal relationship with others and interpersonal communication, users discuss about their "real-self" through social networking. But the ill-assorted thing is that face to face interaction is decreased because of the rise in social networking. **Ramaley, J. A., & Zia, L. (2005)** the students "need for immediacy" is satisfied through social networking. **Notley, T., & Tacchi, J. (2005)** sense of distinctiveness, creativeness and community is developed because of social networking. **Jackson, L. A., et al (2006)** found positive impact in social networking as reading skills, grades improved in the social networking students. **Ito, M., & Okabe, D. (2005), Boase, J., & Wellman, B. (2006), Burns, E. (2007), Richardson, I., et al (2007)** noted, improved connectedness, self-efficacy, knowledge and mental wellbeing among social networking users. **Jenkins, H. (2007)** knowledge and skill is enhanced by using social networking. **Munt, S. R., et al 2002, Hillier, L., & Harrison, L. (2007)** suggested that sense of belonging is fostered through social networking.

Blanchard, M., et al (2007) affirmed, social networking boosts the confidence level, relation between instructors and their scholars. **Ellison, N. S., et al (2007)** pointed out that new relation is formed and existing relation is continued in social networking. **Boyd, D. (2007)** made it clear that, socialisation is indispensable for the psychosocial advance of adolescents and social networking paves a way for it. **Bessière, K., et al (2008)** specified that positive attitude is created in adults through social networking. **Neelamalar, M., & Chitra, P. (2009)** found in their study on social networking among young citizens of India that social networking helps in increasing the knowledge level, connecting people, building friendship and relations. **Mazer, J. P., et al (2009)** guaranteed that relation between teachers and students can be promoted through social networking. **Bonetti, L., et al (2010)** focussed that identity is revealed, rapport is established and friendship blooms through social networking. **Brady, K. P., et al (2010)** studied the benefits of social networking; case study on the benefits of online learning projected the positive aspects of social networking in higher education field. **Lenhart, A., et al (2010)** stated that social networking promotes independence, freedom to communicate, socially interact and seek social support. **Dickson, A., & Holley, R. P. (2010)** researched the academic utilize of social networking between pupils and educators in USA, settled that social networking has affirmative effect in education.

Greenhow, C. (2011) social networking creates learning place for the younger generation, helps in doing school related works and academic stress is reduced through social networking. **Chen, Y. J., et al (2014)** found that general internet use has an indirect positive effect on student's academic performance, in high school students. **Cole, D. A., et al (2017)** conducted a study in 231 undergraduate students regarding the online support. The study emphasize that by increasing social relations through social networking, it increases the social support system. **Kim, B. (2020)** evaluated the social media and its influence in trauma. The findings revealed that immediate sharing of emotion and resilience occurs through social media in case of loneliness / isolation and in times of psychological trauma. Resilience is promoted through social networking. **Alaslani, K., & Alandejani, M. (2020)** pointed out the social networking factors, pattern and impacts through an exploratory case study among 364 adolescents, Dhahran. The study identified WhatsApp as the preferred site (29.86%), followed by Facebook (21.3%). 49.7% started engaging in social networking sites for more than six years. 51.14% had more than 200 friends in social networking. The main purpose of social networking was to connect with friends. Other reasons include knowledge gain, online shopping. The study revealed significant positive outcome of social networking sites on communication / interaction, learning and academic performance.

2.3.2 Negative Impacts of Social Networking

Kraut, R., et al (1998) perceived that increased use of social networking applications is noted among students with academic failure and also loneliness is prevalent among them. **Chou, C., & Hsiao, M. C. (2000)** studied 910 Taiwanese college students from 12 universities to understand the internet addiction and revealed addiction among 54 adolescents, addicts spend triple (thrice) the number of hours online than non-addicts. The researchers identified increased internet use among Taiwanese students, addicted one's informed damaging impacts especially poor sleep and missing / skipping – food / meals; adversely affected the daily routine. Deterioration in physical and mental health is noted due to the prolonged use of internet.

Kubey, R. W., et al (2001) instructed 576 students to report about their social networking / online engagement by filling a questionnaire about the usage, study habits / performance and personality. Increased social networking can cause dependence to social networking, enhances guilty feeling, loss of control; academic failure, sleep issues, and bunking classes. 9.26% students developed social networking dependence. The researchers recognised academic deficiency in 14% and internet dependence in 56% students. **Anderson, C. A., & Bushman, B. J. (2001)** studied the impacts of student's online life in physical, academic and social areas; found impacts in all the aspects and sleep problems were more among the heavy users. Dependence behavior was more seen in males specially prolonged users, symptoms were similar to the features of drug dependence. Thus the study found surfing as the most common activity among youngsters and proved that social networking can lead to dependence and negative impacts.

Hakala, P., et al (2002) has done a study to elicit out the pain due to internet use among Finnish students. The students reported neck / shoulder / back pain after the augmented use of internet. **Rotunda, R. J., et al (2003), Jenaro, C., et al (2007)** found that internet addiction influences the sleep pattern. Heavy internet users had increased sleep disturbance. **Chak, K., & Leung, L. (2004)** studied 722 social networking users. The observed fact was-increased social networking increases shyness, free access / unlimited usage can lead to amplified social networking among adults. Extensive usage can land up in addiction. **Thatcher, A., et al (2008)** explored the connection between heavy internet use and academic problems among 1399 users using standardised questionnaire. The study found strong positive relation between the variables as heavy internet use can lead to procrastination of assignments, works and studies. This will affect the individual negatively.

Cheever, J. (2009) pointed out the indicators of social networking addiction and listed sleep reduction as the main indicator. When a person spend more time in social networking, it will decrease the sleep and tension builds up, day time drowsiness will be present and may not be able to concentrate in studies / work. This will lead to addiction. **Malat, J., et al (2010)** established that, due to the excessive social networking bad relations are formed among young individuals. **Muñoz-Rivas, M. J., et al (2010)** analyzed the social networking addiction and associated problems, evaluated the relationship between time consumed in social networking and the variables that lead to addiction and problematic use. 927 female students and 374 male students (N=1301) participated in this study. Internet using students who spend more time in internet showed connection behavior that is controlled by negative reinforcement, behavioral problems when the connection is lost, augmented stimulation when online, health problems and problems in social, family and academic areas. **Kuppuswamy, S., & Narayan, P. S. (2010)** stated that social networking negatively influences the youngsters, diverts attention and concentration from studies, engage in harmful behaviors. They start social networking for fun and to pass time. **Odaci, H. (2011)** explored the relation between engagement in social networking and academics in 398 college students in Turkey. The findings confirmed negative correlation between academics and internet use related problems.

Kuss, D. J., & Griffiths, M. D. (2011)., Tonioni, F., et al (2012) conveyed negative concerns due to social networking in adolescents. **Yadav, P., et al (2013)** has done a study among 11th and 12th standard students in India, related to their online addiction. Among 552 respondents, 179 (32%) reported their academic performance level as excellent / good, 373 (68%) reported it as average / poor. The study found no association between the variables. The study found positive correlation between addiction in internet and depression, anxiety, stress. **Kwan, G. C. E., & Skoric, M.M. (2013)** explored bullying in social networking among 1676 adolescent students (13 -17 years). The study discovered that 59.4% (n = 1493) were victims of bullying. Sending disgusting / threatening messages, being affronted frequently, being omitted from groups / tricked into revealing secrets, masquerading as someone different, threatening others and hacking account were the bullying incidents happened. The negative impacts of social networking ruled out in this study were physical, psychological, interpersonal, and behavioral problem.

Alam, S. S., et al (2014) explored the harmful side of social networking among 200 teenagers, Malaysia. **Odacı, H., & Çıkrıkçı, Ö. (2014)** observed and studied the internet use related issues among 398 collegiate students. The study identified the cause of poor well-being as problematic internet use. **Vernon, L., et al (2015)** has taken 1886 adolescent students to find out the social networking in the school. The investigation identified – heavy social networking, use increased sleep problems and poor school experience. **Owusu-Acheaw, M., & Larson, A. G. (2015)** performed a study on social networking and academics, among 200 students, Ghana. Only few respondents did not own mobile phones with internet facility, the time spend in social networking daily was thirty minutes to three hours. Increased social networking users were showing poor performance academically. **Rücker, J., et al (2015)** identified the relationship between awkward internet use and substance abuse in 3067 adolescents, Switzerland using internet addiction test. The study findings conclude that risky behavior develops due to excessive social networking / internet use. **Mohammadi, M., et al (2015)** explored the relation between use of internet and education. The study was done among 380 collegiate students. Positive connection was found between internet use and procrastination of academic work.

Kootesh, B. R., et al (2016) undertook a correlation study to assess the sleep and mental health of internet users among 250 students. The sleep quality, mental health and addiction in internet were checked with standardized questionnaires. The analysis showed significant positive relationship between internet addiction with mental health and sleep. Physiological problems also arise due to increased social networking. Increased use of internet will reduce the sleep and cause depression. **Ye, Y. L., et al (2016)** checked the association between compound wellbeing risk issues and mental health among 2422 students, China. The occurrence of sleep problems, nutritional problems, internet addiction, use of alcohol and smoking was 42.6, 29.8, 22.3, 11.6 and 9.3%, respectively. The study also showed increased anxiety and depression.

Seabrook, E. M. (2016) conducted a review on social networking and the related psychiatric outcome-anxiety and depression. Out of the 302 full-text articles revised, 15 articles showed the beneficial and destructive facets of mental health. 70 articles contain depression / anxiety / well-being. 22 studies highlighted depression / anxiety as the significant probable moderators / mediators in social networking with respect to mental health. Out of 30 studies, in 8 readings- a straight positive association was found with depression and noted direct positive association with anxiety in 3 studies. **Younes, F., et al (2016)** assessed 600 college students; the addiction in social networking and its relation with poor sleep, apprehension, depression, tension and self-confidence. The study found correlation between addiction in social networking and poor sleep, apprehension, depression, tension and self-confidence. **Toker, S., & Baturay, M. H. (2016)** focused a research on the effect of game addiction in 159 students doing under graduation. The study proved that game addiction decreases academic performance.

Verduyn, P., et al (2017) checked the detrimental effects of social networking. The study found positive relationship between social networking (active) and well-being, negative relationship between social networking (passive) and well-being. **Rosenkranz, T., et al (2017)** identified the potential for addiction among 5667 adolescents. Chatting was more among girls, gaming was more in social networking boys. Problematic gamers showed many problems than other gamers. **Abdullatif, A.M., et al (2017)** has conducted an investigation on the incorporation of social networking for communication, academic purpose by the technology and academical staff, Saudi University. The study identified some of the major problems faced due to social networking-wastage of time, privacy issues, data security, cyber-bullying etc. **Calancie, O., et al (2017)** analysed the social networking stressors and anxiety among adolescents qualitatively. Some of the samples mentioned fear related to the negative comments online, positive emotions due to the "likes", reported increased anxiety when they compared with others on Facebook. Thus the study strongly underlines that Facebook aggravates anxiety in clients with anxiety disorder and increases chances for negative online experience.

Moqbel, M., & Kock, N. (2018) analysed the personal, job impacts of social networking through 276 questionnaires from technology corporation employees. The results underline that social networking addiction has negative impacts on personal and job area. **Zhang, Y., et al (2018)** focused a study regarding the association between academics and social networking addiction in 2407 students. The results highly stressed that social networking addiction leads to poor educational performance and their by poor academic achievement. **Van Den Eijnden, R., et al (2018)** studied the after effect of increased usage of social networking among the 12-15 year old teenagers. Decreased satisfaction in life, poor academic achievement is related to increased engagement in social networking. **Wang, J. L., et al (2018)** lead a study among 350 college students from China. The study assessed the social networking usage and wellbeing. The study outcome showed poor wellbeing among the heavy social networking users. **Giunchiglia, F., et al (2018)** identified that negative impacts occur due to social networking on academics.

Sampasa-Kanyinga, H., et al (2018) identified the relation between sleep and social networking among 5242 students (11-20 years) in Canada. One hour in social networking is spent by 73.4% students, reduced sleep was present among 63.6% and increased sleep was present in 36.4%. The study concluded that increased social networking is related to decreased sleep. **Martínez-Ferrer, B., et al (2018)** discovered problematic use of social networking among 11-16 year old adolescents. The 1952 respondents were selected through randomized cluster sampling from the secondary schools, Spain. The study findings revealed significant positive relationship between increased social networking and aggressive tendency. Aggression is related to increased impulsivity and poor impulse control. Adjustment problems arise due to excessive social networking. Excessive social networking was noted among adolescent girls.

Grubbs, J. B., et al (2018) calculated the relationship between pornography and social networking addiction, found association between both. **Masthi, N. R., et al (2018)** compared the social networking and health among the students in an urban college, Bangalore. The addictive behavior among the 1870 students was checked with the help of a tool developed by the researchers. Multistage sampling was selected for the study. 36.9% was addicted to social networking. Eye strain (38.4%), anger (25.5%), decreased sleep (26.1%), neck pain (30.7%), gastritis (1.9%) and ring anxiety (66%) was noted among the social networking users. **Kojima, R., et al (2019)** identified the problematic internet use and the impact on health. From 2014-2016, three consecutive survey was done among the students in high school. 979, 968, 940 students were assessed respectively. 19.9% was the prevalence in 2014, 15.9% in 2015 and 17.7% in 2016. Skipping breakfast / meals, late bedtime, drowsiness in the morning, not able to study and features of depression were more among the heavy users. **Tafesse, W. (2020)** evaluated the role of social networking in student's education among 180 collegiate students. The study found negative association between academics and social networking.

2.3.3 Positive and Negative Impacts of Social Networking

Best, P., et al (2014) reported increased wellbeing and cyber bullying; noted after social networking. Social networking has both positive and negative effect. **Parvathy, J., & Suchithra, R. (2015)** studied, "Impact of Usage of Social Networking Sites on Youth". Data collected from 150 respondents through structured questionnaire. Non Probability method of sample selection was used for this study, convenience sampling technique. This study winded with projecting the helpful and damaging aspects of social networking. **Yoo, J. H., & Jeong, E. J. (2017)** checked the effect of social networking use on psychosocial wellbeing (depression, loneliness and life satisfaction). The study shows that use of social networking increased the rate of depression, the network size. The increased network size enhanced the degree of life satisfaction. **Kim, S. Y., et al (2017)** has obtained cross sectional data from 2013 adolescents regarding the association between performance in education and online behavior. Academic performance was correlated positively on the basis of study purpose of social networking and adversely correlated with common purpose.

Bhardwaj, A., et al (2017) explored the consequence of social networking among teenagers, India. The researchers found from the study that social networking has both bright and dark side. Social networking helps in learning, gaining information, increased communication and relationship. The negative aspects include poor academic performance, invasion of privacy, hacking and time waste. Threatening others can cause mental trauma in victims and can lead to suicide. Anxiety, depression and loneliness are the other mental health problems due to social networking. **Harrath, Y., & Alobaidy, H. (2018)** directed a survey through internet regarding the social networking impacts on academic performance among six hundred and twenty eight college students in Bahrain. The study projected out that social networking has both constructive and harmful effects on educational performance. **Vermeulen, A., et al (2018)** interviewed 22 adolescents in-depth regarding the use of multiple social media platforms. Through Facebook, Instagram, and Snap chat positive emotions are shared; whereas negative emotions are shared through Twitter and Messenger. **Alejandrino, M. P. R., et al (2018)** surveyed the influence of social networking on studies among the 150 high school students. The survey findings revealed good study habits and increased social media addiction among the students. Thus the study found relationship between the social media addiction and the study habits. **Weinstein, E. (2018)** assessed the constructive and destructive face of social media. The positive impacts of social networking sites include connectedness / closeness, inspiration and fun. The negative impacts include disconnectedness, boredom, distress and envying.

2.4 SOCIAL NETWORKING ADDICTION

Jang, K. S., et al (2008) aimed to spot the factors associated with internet addiction and the mental health symptoms in Korean adolescents. Boys and girls

(N = 912) in the 7th-12th standards of South Korea schools were the samples. Internet-Related Addiction Scale was used as tool. Out of the 851 students, 30% had mild addiction, 4.3% had severe addiction. Male sex, conversation, and lengthier social networking were significantly associated with severe addiction. **Young, K. S. (2008)** classified five types of addiction-game, cybersex, online shopping, cyber relationship and web-surfing addiction. Addicts showed decreased real life interaction and poor academic performance. **Chang, M. K., & Law, S. P. M. (2008)** assessed "the internet addiction test" by Young, with the help of responses from 410 undergraduates, Hongkong University. Factor analysis was done. The assessment finding proved that the performance of the students-academically was negatively correlated with addiction on internet. High score in internet addiction test was noted among undergraduates with cyber relationships, online gambling.

Choi, K., et al (2009) examined 2336 Korean high school students, their social networking and sleep pattern. 2.5% of addicts were boys, 53.7% of the boys were showing features that can lead to addiction; whereas 1.9% of girls were addicts and 38.9% were showing features that can lead to internet / social networking addiction. Sleep problems were more among the addicts. These include bruxism, decreased sleep, scaring dreams etc. **Young, K. (2009)** focused a study on social networking addiction. The study revealed features of addiction such as carelessness of individual life, preoccupation, escapism and tolerance among the heavy users. **Huang, R. L., et al (2009)** investigated the prevalence and factors of challenging internet use among 3496 university students. 9.58% (boys 13.54%, girls 4.88%) of the students had problematic engagement online. Reduced educational accomplishment, absence of affection from the family was the factors that found to be significantly associated with unhealthy use and these factors are predictors of increased online engagement. About 48.51% were mild users (5 hours / week), 16.36% students were hefty users (>15 hours / week). 25.53% of the students with sadness had features of problematic use. Correlation was noted between depression and problematic use.

Mentzoni, R. A., et al (2011) estimated the rate of extensive involvement in gaming, addiction and its relationship with health status-both physical and psychological. Out of 2500 people, 816 responded to the questionnaire. The investigation identified that problematic video game users had less life satisfaction and reported high level of anxiety, depression. 56.3% were regular video game users, 0.6% were having addiction, 4.1% were problematic users of video game. **Durocher, J. J., et al (2011)** implemented a research on internet usage among 21 college students of age 18 to 23 years. They disclosed that when one cannot access internet, it leads to anxiety and further increases the blood pressure and makes the individual at risk for cardio vascular diseases. **Jain, M. R., et al (2012)** discovered the impact of social networking; males devote extra time than females in social networking and once they log out, the adolescents were thinking of engaging in social networking.

Durkee, T., et al (2012) identified maladaptive and pathologic internet use through a cross-sectional survey in adolescents from 11 countries. The problematic internet use was more seen in males, they used internet mainly for watching videos, chatting; increased online gaming was found in males and social networking in females. Adolescents in urban areas, not staying with parents, lesser involvement of parents and parental joblessness was associated with problematic and maladaptive internet use. The use was pathologic among 4.4% adolescents; increased risk was found among those youngsters who lack support emotionally. **Lee, Y. S., et al (2013)** evaluated the internet addiction among 73238 adolescents studying in middle and high school, South Korea. 3.0% adolescents in the study were at high risk for internet addiction, 11.9% were having possible risk for addiction and 85.2% were normal users. Students with internet addiction were prone for behavioral problems, depression and anxiety. **Niculović, M., et al (2014)** studied pathologic internet use, behavior and attitudes among university students, Belgrade. Pathological symptoms of addiction were noticed among 47.6% students, 46.4% students were less addicted and 6% had no symptoms of addiction. The study revealed strong difference between severely addicted and less addicted students with regard to relationship and personality.

Tsitsika, A., et al (2014) has done a survey to identify the addictive behavior and dysfunctional behavior due to internet among 13,284 school students from seven countries. The study identified that dysfunctional internet behavior was more among boys and differed from country to country. Students who engaged more in gaming, gambling and social networking showed dysfunctional internet behavior (DIB). This behavior was more among boys and it differed from country to country. Through multiple logistic regression analysis, it was clear that this behavior was more among students of parents with low level of education, students who engage more in gaming, social networking and those who started using internet at a very early age. **Hormes, J. M., et al (2014)** performed a survey among 253 college students, to catch out the association between social networking addiction and behavior. Tool used include disordered online social networking use, DSM-IV-TR diagnostic criteria for dependence and Young Internet Addiction Test. Increased usage was found in 9.7% and they reported various features of addiction such as tolerance / need more time in social networking and withdrawal / irritation / anger, when unable to access the social networking.

Loton, D., et al (2016) analysed the effect of game addiction on mental health. There were 552 adults, as participants from Australia. Standardized tools used for the online survey include addiction, anxiety, depression and coping. From the study it was obvious that there was relationship between game addiction and apprehension, depression, stress. **McNicol, M. L., & Thorsteinsson, E. B. (2017)** investigated addiction on internet, mental distress and coping among 449 youths. Data analysis revealed 68.9% teenagers were without problematic use, 24.4% with problematic use and 6.7% with addiction. Low self-care was observed in addicts. Predictors of addiction in internet include online sex, online gaming and anxiety. **Bargeron, A. H., & Hormes, J. M. (2017)** has done a study on psychosocial associates of gaming disorder, based on DSM-5 criteria. The samples who met the criteria for internet gaming disorder reported more symptoms of psychosocial dysfunction, depression, apprehension, stress, lower life gratification and increased impulsivity. **Seabra, L., et al (2017)** focused on self-esteem and online addiction with the help of Internet Addiction Test (IAT) - Young, K. (1998b), Rosenberg Self-Esteem Scale (RSES) - Rosenberg, M. (1989) among 1399 users, Brazil. The study underlines negative correlation between self-esteem and online addiction. That is higher the internet addiction, lower will be the self-esteem. Negative emotions evident in internet addicts were sadness, irritability, and distress; this leads to decreased self-esteem.

Basu, S., et al (2018) explored the features of addiction in increased mobile phone use through a cross sectional study among 233 medical undergraduates, India. The participants belongs to the adolescent group (10-19 years). 74% of the students used mobile for surfing, 66.1% used for messaging and 64.8% used it for social networking. 26.4% reported that, they are not able to concentrate. 39.9% had mobile phone addiction; while 60.1% students were free from mobile phone addiction. The study identified destructive use, strong craving, poor control, and tolerance as the features of mobile phone addiction. **Jogi, M. S., et al (2018)** scrutinised the occurrence and aspects associated with social networking addiction. The samples included in the study were 120 middle adolescents in standard X and XII studying in a higher secondary school at Kashmir and the sampling method was simple random. The results projected out that 20.8% student were showing dependence to social networking. No significant association of social networking with sex and socio economic profile; while noteworthy relationship exists with residence.

Kayastha, B., et al (2018) measured internet addiction and its impact by doing a descriptive research. The samples were 200 high school students, in Mangalore, India. The study made known that 70.5% were normal users, 23% were addicted mildly, 6% were addicted moderately and 0.5% had severe addiction. The impact of internet was mild among 73%, moderate among 16.5% and 10.5% of samples had no impact. **Chacón-Borrego, F., et al (2018)** examined the intra / interpersonal addiction due to problematic internet use, association between dependence, cyber bullying and physical activity through a non-experimental study among 184 higher secondary students. The study results stressed that there is a need of continuously checking the social networking and WhatsApp; internet is used in order to escape from problems and to withdraw from other engagements. The study also found a relation between the internet addiction and cyber bullying.

2.5 SOCIAL NETWORKING AND MENTAL HEALTH

Davis, R. A., et al (2002) administered 325 forms to psychology undergraduate students in a university, Canada. The dangerous effects of internet use were assessed among 211 participants; sadness, isolation and postponement of work were associated with heavy / problematic engagement. **Pantic, I., et al (2012)** observed the high school students and studied the associates between social networking and depression, identified noteworthy correlation between depression and time spend in social networking. **Blomfield Neira, C. J., & Barber, B. L. (2014)** examined the association between depression and social networking among 1,819 high school students. The findings proved that social networking is related to decreased confidence and low mood. **Harwood, J., et al (2014)** studied the after effect (mental health changes) of increased use of internet for browsing, texting, gaming, mailing, social networking and making calls. Survey was done through online among 274 people using various questionnaires on demographic details, use of smart phone, internet addiction and mental health assessment. From the study it was identified that increased social networking has led to increased level of stress and depression.

Bezinović, P., et al (2015) compared the pattern of internet use and mental health variables in 1539 students in a high school, Croatia. The key features identified through the study were: boys were problematic users and had aggression. Girls experienced harassment, had ill health, sadness and felt lonely. The students accessed social networking for the purpose of enjoyment and interaction. **Rohilla, P. S., & Kumar, K. (2015)** identified a link between social networking and psychiatric problems in the adults. Mental health problems include anxiety, depression, loneliness, compulsive behavior. **Malliga, T. (2015)** assessed the consequence of social networking on mental health and academic achievement among middle adolescents, TamilNadu, India. The study showed significant difference between boys and girls, no significant difference between the living place - rural and urban students, no significant difference between the aided and unaided school students, no significant difference between owning computer / mobile phone and no significant difference between the social networking impact on mental health and academics.

Seabrook, E. M. (2016) reviewed and summarized research examining depression and anxiety among social networking users. The study concluded that depression and anxiety is reduced due to the positive bond, care and interactions; it has increased the satisfaction of people, confidence in them. In case of negative impact, interaction anxiety and depressive symptoms can aggravate. **Woods, H. C., & Scott, H. (2016)** studied the impact of social media, social networking among 467 youngsters. The study revealed that social networking leads to reduced sleep, self-esteem, depression and anxiety. **Wu, X. S., et al (2016)** has done a cross sectional study to evaluate internet addiction among 10158 adolescents from China. Standardized questionnaires were used for this study. From the study it was noted that control of parents, income of parents, performance in studies, internet accessibility, activities engaged in online has effects on addiction due to internet. Internet addiction was less among people who had social support. 10.4% was the prevalence rate of addiction. A major finding of the study was depression, note among internet addicted people.

Donnelly, E., & Kuss, D. J. (2016) performed an online cross sectional study; examined the increased social networking and depressive features / addiction among the 103 social networking users. The findings indicated that the main predictor of depression is social networking addiction. The youngsters who spend augmented time in social networking had addictive symptoms. Through the model developed in the study, it was proved that increased social networking usage and social networking addiction will predict depression; social networking addiction will mediate depression. **Choi, T. R., et al (2017)** has done an investigation to interpret the relation of mental health and internet use through self-reported questionnaire from 1248 school students, Korea. The study proved correlation between mental health and internet use. **Kim, H. H. S. (2017)** performed a longitudinal cohort study on social networking impacts among 2844 Korean students. The researcher identified that increased engagement in front of the computer screen is linked with mental health problems. Cyber bullying increases the suicidal tendency, those who have good parental support can prevent this. Academic stress can also cause poor mental wellbeing. Strong, negative relationship was noted between chatting, e-mailing and mental health, suicidal ideation.

Pontes, H. M. (2017) conducted a study regarding the entertainment affinity in social networking among 700 middle school students from Portugal. Depression and anxiety was assessed in order to examine their mental wellbeing. Structural equation modeling showed that depression and anxiety arises out of social networking addiction. Increased social networking for entertainment purpose will make the adolescents addicted to social networking. **Berryman, C., et al (2018)** examined the after effect of social media through a correlation study among 467 youngsters. The results indicate that social networking is not a predictor of mental wellbeing. **Barman, L., et al (2018)** examined the prevalence and pattern of social networking and associated psychiatric problems in youngsters, West Bengal. The study was cross-sectional, sample size was 200. The study concluded that more than 90% of the teenagers are active in many social networking sites, 80% engaged it more than 4 hours per day, 55% engage in odd timings, 23.5% showed features of craving (not able to spend even a day without social networking). 24% of the respondents noticed depression and 68.5% had anxiety.

Kitazawa, M., et al (2018) has done a survey to find out the negative impacts of internet use among 1336 samples (young adults), Japan. Females were showing more internet use in a problematic manner. Problematic users used the internet longer, had poor sleep, increased features of depression and anxiety. **Reinecke, L., et al (2018)** assessed the relation between internet use, procrastination and mental wellbeing. The sample size was 1577. The German people who use internet were included for the study. The study revealed that people with trait procrastination had failure in controlling the excess use of internet, identified correlation with regard to stress, anxiety, depression. Thus it was proved that social networking is a reason for the delay in task. **Hussain, Z., & Griffiths, M. D. (2018)** has done a cross-sectional survey, analysed the association between the challenging social networking and mental illness. The review of latest studies found that problematic social networking was related with depressive features, symptoms of anxiety and stress. The social networking excess is highly related to depression and anxiety. **Abdul Ghani, W. S. W., et al (2019)** found out the relation between social networking addiction and mental health problems. The survey was done among 61participants, using structured questionnaire. The researchers concluded that anxiety, depression arise because of social networking addiction.

Kim, M. H., et al (2019) performed an online survey on use of smart phone and associated issues among 62,276, 12-18 years old adolescents, Korea. The findings indicate keener phone use among girls, city residents, middle / low socio-economic status, students with poor sleep and increased stress. The use of smart phone was for learning purpose, information gaining, playing online games, viewing a movie, hearing music and online shopping; that is process purpose. Social purpose of smart phone includes chatting and social networking. Process purpose had strong association with negative impacts; while moderate use for social purpose revealed certain protection against suicide attempt. Among the students who spend more time in phone; conflict, poor academic performance and suicidal attempt was observed. Conflict causes poor relationship and poor mental health. **Saikia et al (2019)** assessed the internet addiction, social networking through a cross-sectional design among the 440 higher secondary students, Assam, India. The prevalence of addiction was mild addiction - 65.4%, moderate addiction - 13.46% and severe addiction 1.9%. The main reason behind internet use was for social networking (71.4%) and for study (42.1%). The study noted significant association between internet addiction and stress, anxiety, depression. Prevalence of depression was found among the 85.7% students and anxiety among the 83.3% students.

Kircaburun, K., et al (2019) performed a detailed study on the problematic social networking among the 470 teenagers. The study projected out positive association between depression and problematic social networking. **Emirtekin, E., et al (2019)** conducted a research on problematic smart phone use among 443 adolescents. The study found association between anxiety, depression and problematic smart phone use. **Li, X., et al (2019)** examined 1545 youngsters and studied the association between anxiety, depression, sex, obesity, and social networking addiction. The study was done in China, revealed increased addiction in males and anxiety is associated with social networking addiction. **Vahedi, Z., & Zannella, L. (2019)** have done a meta-analysis to rule out whether there exists a relation between social networking and depression. The findings revealed association between social networking and depression.

Hussain, Z., et al (2020) reviewed 35 studies related to social networking, its psychological impacts through various data base. Ten studies with association between social networking and anxiety, depression was identified. **Jenkins, R. H., et al (2020)** evaluated the social networking usage and quality of life, behavior among 5229 adolescents. The study found increased social networking among the participants and it is associated with poor quality of life and increased behavioral issues. Excessive night awakening for social networking leads to decreased quality of life and greater behavioral problems. **Abi-Jaoude, E., et al (2020)** explored the relation between social networking, smart phone use and mental health. The researchers identified that social networking increases a sense of community and belongingness. Social networking addiction can lead to poor mental wellbeing and suicidal tendency. Poor sleep can act as a mediator in night time social networking and low mood. **Balcerowska, J. M., et al (2020)** explored social networking addiction and its relation with mental health among 1099 teenagers. The personality, stress, social networking addiction and wellbeing was assessed with the standardised questionnaires. Social networking addiction was inversely associated with emotional steadiness, negatively associated with wellbeing.

2.6 SUMMARY

The present review of literature is a blue print that shows the influence of technology, specifically social networking and its impacts among the users. Social networking fascinates and attracts the adolescents; motivate them to explore their areas of interest. Low cost, simplicity, and increased features create temptation to utilize social networking widely. It is used increasingly and excessively mainly for entertainment, gaining information, online shopping and to interact with others. Social networking has positive impacts on mental health like increased sense of belongingness, communication, escapism from unpleasant situations, sense of identity, empowerment, attachment, accomplishment, encouragement, support, connectedness, interaction, decreased anxiety, increased leadership, psychological wellbeing and socialization. The consequence is elaborated under negative impacts, that mainly include physical, academic, psychological, adjustment and familial impacts.

CHAPTER 3

RESEARCH METHODOLOGY

3.1 INTRODUCTION

The present chapter comprises of the methods followed in the study which includes detailed description of the research design utilized; formulated hypotheses and the variables of the study. A portrayal of the samples, sample size, setting has been included and elucidation of the questionnaires used to gather the quantitative data of the study is clearly depicted. Discussion is done on the procedure and methods followed in order to carry out both the quantitative as well as qualitative aspects of the study.

3.2 RESEARCH DESIGN

Sequential Explanatory Mixed Method design, which includes both quantitative and qualitative analyses, was adopted for the present study. This mixed method helps in identifying the extent of social networking, depicts a blueprint on the purposes of social networking, its impacts on humane and the extent of behavioral changes. Quantitative research was conducted with the help of questionnaire and qualitative study with the help of semi-structured in-depth interviews. Quantitative and qualitative data findings were incorporated jointly in the results of the study.

3.2.1 Sequential Explanatory Mixed Method Approach

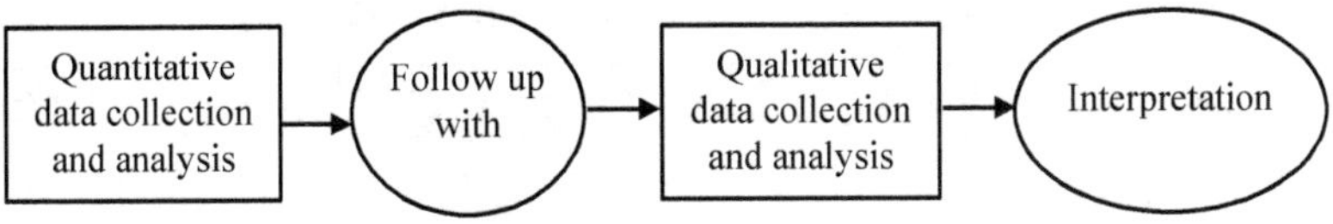

Figure 3.1 Sequential Explanatory Mixed Method Approach

Two types of information can be gained by collecting sequential quantitative and qualitative data, helps in better understanding the topic, Bowen, P., et al (2017).

3.2.2 Overview of Research Process

Table 3.1 Overview of Research Process

Design of the study	Sequential Explanatory Design
Theoretical paradigm	Quantitative study Qualitative study
Methodology	Explanatory sequential method.
Participants	Middle adolescents: 15-17 years (WHO, AAP) Std X, XI, XII
Data collection technique	Quantitative (Questionnaire) Qualitative (Interviews)
Ethics	Permission obtained from the Directorate of General Education, school authorities. Consent taken from students and their parents.
Data analysis	SPSS 20 AMOS 24 NVIVO 12
Validity, reliability	Face validity, Cronbach's alpha

Source: Adapted from Bryman, A., & Cramer, D. (2004). Bowen, P., et al (2017)

3.2.3 Phases of Research

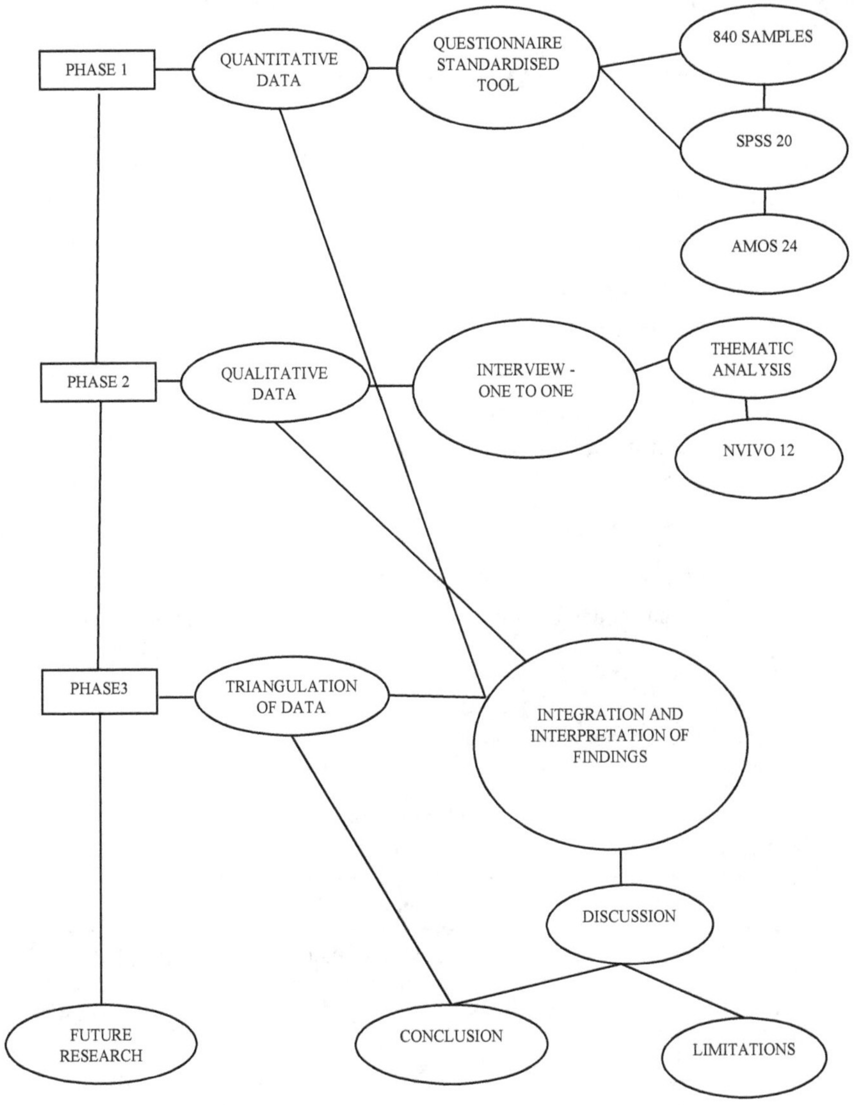

Figure 3.2 Phases of Research

3.3 PERIOD OF STUDY

The total duration of the study was four years (2017-2021).

3.4 SAMPLING FRAMEWORK

After seeking approval from The Directorate of General Education (Annexure IV), screening of government, aided and unaided schools under the Kerala State Board was carried out. Schools in the Trivandrum Corporation was 84. Out of the 84 schools identified, through random number generator (RAO software) method four schools from government sector, three schools from aided sector and two schools from unaided sector were selected for the study.

3.5 SAMPLING TECHNIQUE

A random sample of students from middle adolescent age group ranging 15 to 17 years (WHO, AAP), studying in standard X to XII was drawn from Thiruvananthapuram District, Kerala state following stratified random sampling method.

3.5.1 Description of Samples

Table 3.2 Description of Samples

School												Grand Total
Government					Aided				Unaided			
1	2	3	4	Total	1	2	3	Total	1	2	Total	
25	25	25	24	99	33	33	33	99	49	49	98	296
25	25	25	24	99	33	33	33	99	49	49	98	296
24	24	24	24	96	32	32	32	96	48	48	96	288
												880

Source: Primary data

3.6 SAMPLING METHOD

The subjects of the study were chosen based on the inclusion and exclusion criteria.

3.6.1 Inclusion Criteria

- Adolescent student social networking users of age 15 to 17 years and those who were in Std X, XI and XII.
- Students who got parental consent, voluntarily agreed to participate.
- Students in English medium, those who can read, speak and write English.
- Students those who study in Kerala state syllabus.

3.6.2 Exclusion Criteria

- Students of age other than 15 to 17 years.
- Students who hesitate to participate.
- Students who never used social networking gadgets.
- Students with intellectual difficulties, deaf, dump and visually challenged.

3.7 SAMPLE SIZE DETERMINATION

The sample consists of 840 middle adolescent students consisting of 420 males and 420 females. The students come from varying ethnic backgrounds. The age of the participants ranging from 15 to 17 years, studying in standard X, XI, XII at different sectors of schools such as government, aided and unaided sector in Trivandrum district, Kerala state (Epi Info is Epi Info 7-Epidemiological studies). Sample size was calculated based on Goel, D., et al (2013) the prevalence of internet addiction among adolescents -25.5%, with 95% confidence limit and 12% of relative precision, estimated using the following formula.

Formula for sample size estimation = $(z)^2 x (1-p) / (p) x (e)^2$

Sample size (N) = $(1.96)^2 x (1-0.255) / 0\ 255x (0.12)^2$

= 3.84(0.745) / 0.003672

= 780. Samples needed was 780, but 100 samples were taken extra (880), after removing the incomplete data samples, 840 were included in the study.

3.8 SCALE DEVELOPMENT

The present study focuses on the mental health of middle adolescent student (15 to 17 years) social networking users. Tools used for the study were socio demographic profile, social networking inventory and mental health questionnaire. The two major variables of the study are as follows:

3.8.1 Variables

3.8.1.1 Social Networking

Social networking is defined as the behavior involved in using online platforms / sites / application for various purposes like relationship building, gaining knowledge, entertainment and to purchase things online. The variables including age of starting social networking, preferred social networking sites, preferred usage time (day or night), type of device, preferred place for social networking, preferred area of interest, type of friends in social networking, reasons for social networking, various impacts and addiction was assessed.

3.8.1.2 Mental Health

Mental health refers to feeling good, optimistic, confident, think clearly and able to solve problems. Positive wellbeing after engaging in social networking is assessed.

3.9 PILOT STUDY

A pilot study was done among 60 middle adolescent students studying in government, aided and unaided schools in Trivandrum Corporation, to explore the feasibility of the study and tool development. It was observed that a good rapport needs to be established with the school authorities to meet the participants. There was a need for good supervision; clarification. An average of 15 minutes time was taken by each student to complete the questionnaire. The data obtained from the pilot study was analyzed for the tool development. The reliability of the tool was checked after the pilot study, depicted in Table 3.3.

3.9.1 Reliability of the Instrument

Table 3.3 Reliability of the Instrument

Sl No.	Constructs / Variables	Reliability Score
Reasons for Preferring Social Networking: (Ryan, T., & Xenos, S. 2011; Griffiths, M. D., et al 2014; Abbas, J., et al 2019) I engage in social networking because of…..		
1	Low cost	0.947
2	Easy accessibility	0.947
3	Privacy	0.947
4	Satisfaction of need	0.947
5	Curiosity	0.947
6	Worldwide acceptance	0.946
7	Thinking that it is a part of life	0.945
8	Freedom	0.956
9	Feeling that everything is available in internet	0.946
10	Increased interest in using smart phone	0.947
11	Less monitoring of parents	0.947

Sl No.	Constructs / Variables	Reliability Score
12	Poor parent-child relationship	0.947
13	Influence of friends	0.947
14	Escaping S from studies	0.947
15	Opportunity to forget previous bad experience	0.947
16	Lack of interest in hobbies	0.947
17	Lack of life satisfaction	0.945
18	Reducing suicidal thoughts	0.945
19	Fear on face to face interaction	0.944
20	Reducing stress	0.945
21	Reducing nervousness	0.945
22	Excessive web surfing	0.945
23	Interest in sending threatening email, to frighten others	0.945
24	Increased interest in online sex	0.946
Reasons for Social Networking Habit: (Andreassen, C. S. 2015) When I am online, I engage in social networking,		
1	I use it regularly	0.885
2	I think it is time-consuming	0.882
3	I feel anxious, when the network is not available	0.935
4	I repeatedly check phone for messages	0.877
5	I like social networking, because of constant availability	0.876
6	I prefer mobile chat over face to face communication	0.879
7	I feel there is Fear of missing out	0.872
8	I can form my identity	0.875
9	I get social support	0.877

Sl No.	Constructs / Variables	Reliability Score
(Purpose) Reasons for Engaging in Social Networking: (Brandtzæg, P. B., & Heim, J. 2009; Kim, M. H., et al 2019; Karpagam, R., & Loheswari, M., 2020; Kircaburun, K., et al 2020) I engage in social networking …………		
1	To interact with others	0.929
2	To establish and maintain relationship with others	0.917
3	To increase the knowledge level	0.915
4	To have entertainment	0.916
5	To purchase things online	0.929
Importance towards Social Networking (Social Networking Addiction): (Griffiths, M. D. 2018) After engaging in Social networking…………		
1	It became my first priority in life	0.899
2	I neglect all activities	0.898
3	I need more time for it	0.908
4	I face problems	0.906
5	I always think of engaging in it	0.890
6	I wanted to cut down it, but I can't	0.896
7	I get frustrated, when I am not able to access it	0.897
Impacts of Social Networking: (Abbas, J., et al 2019) After engaging in social networking, I used to have…		
Physical Impacts: (Hakala, P., et al 2002; Masthi, N. R., et al 2018)		
1	Pain	0.915
2	Tiredness	0.914
3	Eye problem	0.912
4	Bone problem	0.914
5	Muscle problem	0.909

Sl No.	Constructs / Variables	Reliability Score
6	Breathing problem	0.911
7	Increased heart rate	0.911
8	Decreased sleep	0.930
Academic Impacts: (Giunchiglia, F., et al 2018)		
1	Fear of exams	0.874
2	Fear to answer in the class	0.854
3	Compare with other students	0.927
Psychological Impacts: (Kitazawa, M., et al 2018)		
1	Sadness	0.708
2	Feeling of hopelessness	0.704
3	Feeling of worthlessness	0.702
4	Lack of interest in all activities	0.786
5	No future plan	0.803
6	Substance use	0.815
Impacts on Adjustment: (Martínez-Ferrer, B., et al 2018) After engaging in social networking, I used to……		
1	Get along with others	0.844
2	Conflict with others	0.856
3	Get irritated for simple things	0.839
4	Cry for simple reasons	0.870
Familial Impacts: (Kwan, G. C. E., & Skoric, M. M. 2013)		
1	Conflict among parents	0.822
2	Increased expenditure	0.797
3	Anger towards family members	0.812
4	Steal money from parents	0.866

Source: Primary data

As shown in Table 3.3 after the pilot study, 86 items in the questionnaire was reduced to 70 items, as the sixteen items were with < 0.7 cronbach's alpha.

3.10 PROCESS OF DEVELOPING SOCIAL NETWORKING INVENTORY

The researcher's knowledge, skill and experience in dealing with substance abuse, internet addiction and behavioral issues among adolescents, interaction with Psychiatrists, Psychologists, Psychiatric Social Workers, Epidemiologists and experts from the Department of Education-Kerala Government paved way in the initial stage of developing the questionnaire. The literature review focusing on the socio-demographic data, social networking pattern, factors, reasons, impacts and addictive behaviors contributed to the construction of the first-round questionnaire and item generation.

3.11 FACE VALIDATION, CONTENT VALIDATION

3.11.1 Social Networking Inventory

Under the expert guidance of the research supervisor, first face validation of the items was carried out, along with the doctoral committee members during the doctoral committee meeting. All items derived from the literature were subjected to the process of content validation, done by 23 experts drawn from the field. These experts are listed in the table (Annexure V). Tool was designed to assess the reasons for social networking, addiction and social networking impacts.

3.11.2 Warwick Edinburgh Mental Wellbeing Scale (WEMWBS)

The researchers at the Universities of Warwick and Edinburgh developed the Warwick-Edinburgh Mental Well-being Scale (WEMWBS) in the year 2006. The purpose of this 14 item scale is to assess the mental health of the adolescents.

3.12 DATA COLLECTION METHOD

3.12.1 Quantitative Data

The researcher obtained permission from the Directorate of General Education, Kerala (Annexure IV). School list was issued from the Directorate Office. Nine schools were selected from the list through random number generator. After school selection, permission was taken from the concerned school authorities, Principal / Head master. The investigation was carried out in the year 2019. Consent was taken directly from the parents and students after giving a detailed explanation about the study. They were asked to put signature in the form only if they were willing for the study. The instructions for answering the research tools were read out and explained by the researcher. They were guaranteed of the concealment of their responses and requested to answer all the questions frankly. After that, questionnaire was distributed to them in the following order: Socio demographic tool, Social Networking Inventory and Warwick Edinburgh Mental Wellbeing Scale (WEMWBS) (Annexure I). After completion questionnaires are returned, which were checked for omission and errors.

3.12.2 Qualitative Data

The adolescents who participated in the quantitative study and showed interest in participating in further research were approached for the qualitative study. Among those who were interested (n = 20), semi structured interview was conducted among four adolescents, selected on the basis of the social networking addiction scale scores. The aim of this in-depth semi-structured interview was to extract the views about the purpose of social networking, thoughts and feelings (emotions) when engaged in social networking, perceived benefits and positive impacts of social networking, the problems faced due to social networking and to elicit out whether social networking is a healthy behavior or not. The participants were further probed when detailed information was required based on the obtained responses. They were assured of the confidentiality of their responses, the interview was audio recorded for further analyses. On an average, the interviews extended to about forty five minutes to an hour.

3.13 NORMALITY

An evaluation of the normality of data is a prerequisite, before starting with further analysis in parametric testing. The most widely used methods to test the normality of the data is the Kolmogorov – Smirnov test and the Shapiro – Wilk test. For small sample sizes (<50) Shapiro – Wilk test is more suitable, although it can handle large sample size, Kolmogorov–Smirnov test is used for larger sample size (≥50). P > 0.05 indicates that the data are normally distributed. Normal range for skewness and kurtosis is -2 to +2 (Razali, N. M., & Wah, Y. B. 2011).

Table 3.4 Test of Normality

Dimensions	Kolmogorov-Smirnov[a]			Shapiro-Wilk		
	Statistic	Df	Sig.	Statistic	Df	Sig.
Social Networking Addiction	0.137	840	0.100	0.906	840	0.200
Mental health	0.082	840	0.100	0.966	840	0.200

Source: Primary data

Table 3.4 indicates that the data are normally distributed.

3.14 MEASUREMENT MODEL

3.14.1 Convergent Validity

Convergent validity was evaluated for the three constructs using the three criteria recommended by Fornell & Larcker (1981).

Table 3.5 Average Variance Extracted and Factor Loadings of the Constructs

Construct	Factor Names	Average Variance Extracted	Construct Factor Loadings
1	Social Networking Impacts	0.711	0.84
2	Social Networking Addiction	0.701	0.83
3	Mental Health	0.698	0.82

Source: Primary data

Table 3.5 shows that all the items have high factor loadings; majority of factors have a loading of greater than 0.85. Average variance extracted values are greater than 0.70, well above the requirement of 0.5, demonstrating convergent validity of the model.

3.14.2 Composite Reliability

Reliability, also called consistency and reproducibility, can be defined as the degree to which measurements are free from error and therefore yield consistent results. A value greater than 0.70 reflects a good reliability (Hair et al 2006).

Table 3.6 Composite Reliability and Average Variance Extracted

Constructs	Composite Reliability (CR)	Average Variance Extracted (AVE)
Social Networking Impacts	0.910	0.711
Social Networking Addiction	0.885	0.701
Mental Health	0.974	0.698

Source: Primary data

Table 3.6 shows the composite reliability and average variance extracted of the constructs. The composite reliability for "Mental Health" is found to be 0.974. Similarly, composite reliabilities for other constructs were estimated. All composite reliabilities of the constructs have a value higher than 0.70 (all CR > 0.885) indicating adequate internal consistency of the constructs.

3.14.3 Cronbach's Alpha

Cronbach's alpha is a tool to determine whether the response is consistent. The internal reliability of the measurement models was tested using Fornell's composite reliability (Fornell and Larcker, 1981).

Table 3.7 Cronbach's Alpha for the improved Measurement Model

S No	Constructs	No of Item	Cronbach's Alpha
1	Social Networking Impacts	25	0.960
2	Social Networking Addiction	07	0.855
3	Mental Health	14	0.908

Source: Primary data

Table 3.7 shows that the internal consistency of the scales was high, with Cronbach's alpha values above 0.8 for all the three constructs. Therefore, it is concluded that the responses are consistent.

3.14.4 Discriminant Validity

Discriminant validity is determined by the extent to which a construct is distinct from other constructs. Discriminant validity refers to the extent to which factors are distinct and uncorrelated. The rule is that variables should relate more strongly to their own factor than to another factor. Two primary methods exist for determining discriminant validity. The first method is to examine the pattern matrix. Variables should load significantly only on one factor. If a variable loads on multiple factors, then the cross-loadings should differ by more than 0.2. In this model, the variables have loaded only on one factor.

Table 3.8 Discriminant Validity

	Social Networking Impacts	Mental Health	Social Networking Addiction
Social Networking Impacts	**0.851**		
Mental Health	0.601	**0.895**	
Social Networking Addiction	0.543	0.697	**0.847**

Source: Primary data

Examining the factor correlation matrix from Table 3.8 correlations between factors do not exceed 0.7. A correlation greater than 0.7 is an indication of increased shared variance. As seen from the factor correlation matrix, correlation among the constructs is very low once again confirming discriminant validity.

3.15 CONFIRMING THE MEASUREMENT MODEL

After validating the measurement instrument, the results of the Confirmatory Factor Analysis (CFA) are used to evaluate the model fit of the measurement model. AMOS 24 is used to confirm the hypothesized structure. The measurement model contains all the study factors. Each factor is measured by the observed variables, the reliability of which is influenced by random measurement error, as indicated by the associated error term. Each of these observed variables is regressed into its respective factor. Finally, all the factors are shown to be inter-correlated.

Latent variables are implied by the covariance among two or more measured variables. They are also known as factors (i.e., factor analysis), constructs or unobserved variables. In a measurement model, an arrow is drawn from the measured variable to the constructs. Rectangles or squares are used to indicate measured variables and ellipse or circles represent latent variables. Error terms ("disturbances" for latent variables) are included in the diagram, represented by "E's" for measured variables and "D's" for latent variables. The error terms represent residual variances within variables not accounted for by pathways hypothesized in the model. The hypothesized model is recursive, i.e. Uni-directional. Recursive models are the most straightforward and have two basic features: their disturbances are uncorrelated and all causal effects are unidirectional.

3.15.1 Confirmatory Factor Analysis of Social Networking Impacts

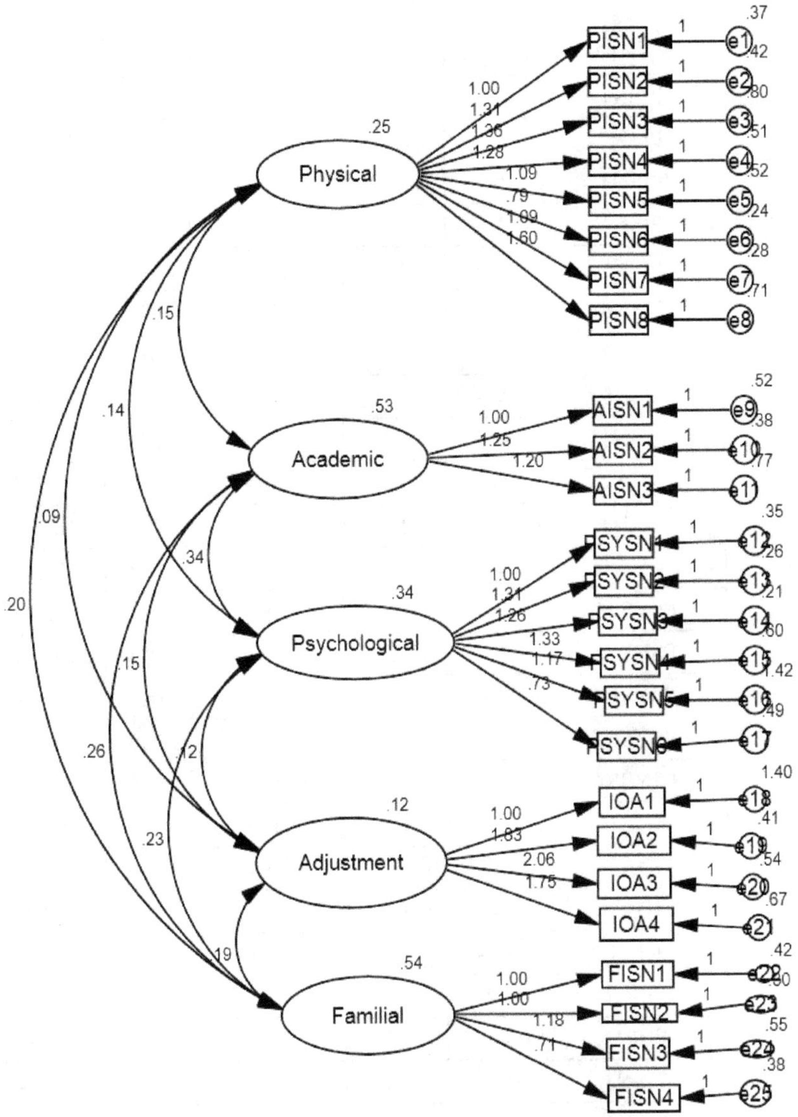

Figure 3.3 Confirmatory Factor Analysis of Social Networking Impacts

Table 3.9 Estimate Table - Confirmatory Factor Analysis of Social Networking Impacts

Social Networking Impacts			Estimate	S.E.	C.R.	P
PISN1	<---	F1	.828	.036	18.763	***
PISN2	<---	F1	.706	.031	18.301	***
PISN3	<---	F1	.704	.034	18.337	***
PISN4	<---	F1	.833	.047	19.144	***
PISN5	<---	F1	.850	.043	18.904	***
PISN6	<---	F1	.709	.044	19.426	***
PISN7	<---	F1	.498	.040	19.426	***
PISN8	<---	F1	.524	.055	19.351	***
AISN1	<---	F3	.710	.034	18.314	***
AISN2	<---	F3	.828	.036	18.763	***
AISN3	<---	F3	.706	.031	18.301	***
PSYSN1	<---	F2	.704	.034	18.337	***
PSYSN2	<---	F2	.497	.032	19.745	***
PSYSN3	<---	F2	.524	.055	19.351	***
PSYSN4	<---	F2	.709	.044	19.426	***
PSYSN5	<---	F2	.498	.040	19.426	***
PSYSN6	<---	F2	.524	.055	19.351	***
IOA1	<---	F4	.279	.044	19.426	***
IOA2	<---	F4	.699	.040	19.351	***
IOA3	<---	F4	.693	.055	19.877	***
IOA4	<---	F4	.593	.055	19.784	***
FISN1	<---	F5	.748	.044	19.039	***
FISN2	<---	F5	.800	.040	18.430	***
FISN3	<---	F5	.759	.055	18.314	***
FISN4	<---	F5	.646	.055	18.763	***

Source: Primary data

3.15.2 Confirmatory Factor Analysis of Social Networking Addiction

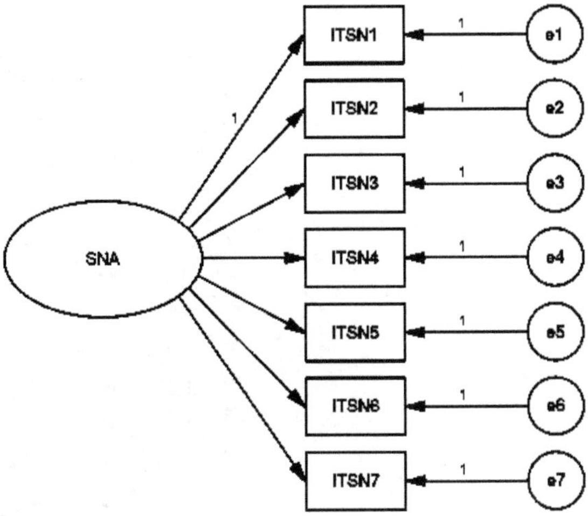

Figure 3.4 Confirmatory Factor Analysis of Social Networking Addiction

Table 3.10 Estimate Table- Confirmatory Factor Analysis of Social Networking Addiction

Social Networking Addiction			Estimate	S.E.	C.R.	P	Label
ITSN1	<---	SNA	1.000				
ITSN2	<---	SNA	1.006	.067	14.997	***	par_1
ITSN3	<---	SNA	1.276	.079	16.087	***	par_2
ITSN4	<---	SNA	1.218	.076	16.057	***	par_3
ITSN5	<---	SNA	1.261	.075	16.734	***	par_4
ITSN6	<---	SNA	1.090	.080	13.684	***	par_5
ITSN7	<---	SNA	1.232	.081	15.218	***	par_6

Source: Primary data

3.15.3 Confirmatory Factor Analysis of Mental Health

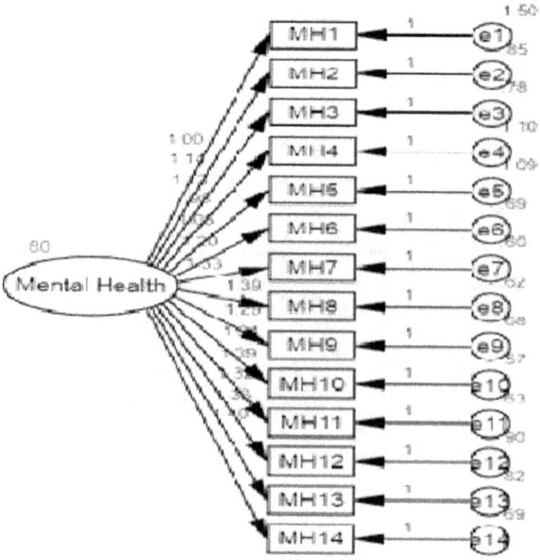

Figure 3.5 Confirmatory Factor analysis of Mental Health

Table 3.21 Estimate Table - Confirmatory Factor Analysis of Mental Health

Mental Health			Estimate	S.E.	C.R.	P
MH1	<---	MH	0.803	0.087	9.258	***
MH2	<---	MH	1.499	0.075	20.019	***
MH3	<---	MH	0.853	0.044	19.426	***
MH4	<---	MH	0.780	0.040	19.351	***
MH5	<---	MH	1.101	0.055	19.877	***
MH6	<---	MH	1.091	0.055	19.784	***
MH7	<---	MH	0.693	0.036	19.039	***
MH8	<---	MH	0.600	0.033	18.430	***
MH9	<---	MH	0.619	0.034	18.314	***
MH10	<---	MH	0.678	0.036	18.763	***
MH11	<---	MH	0.571	0.031	18.301	***
MH12	<---	MH	0.631	0.034	18.337	***
MH13	<---	MH	0.902	0.047	19.144	***
MH14	<---	MH	0.818	0.043	18.904	***

Source: Primary data

3.15.4 Overall Measurement Model

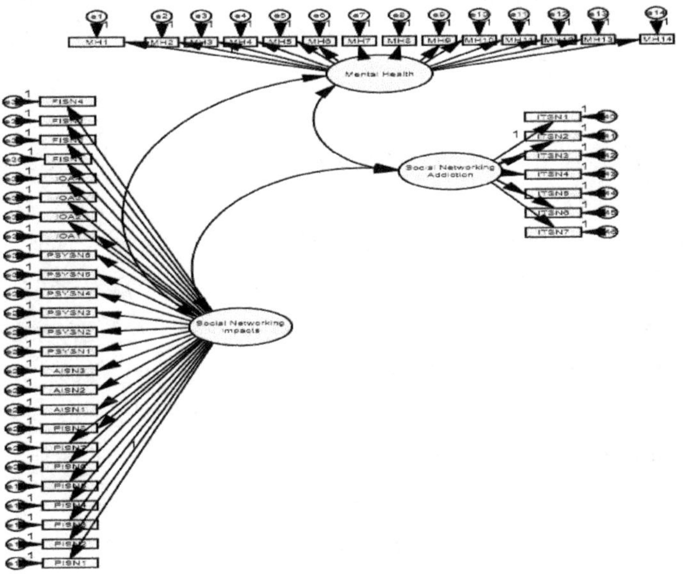

Figure 3.6 Overall Measurement Model

Table 3.12 Confirmatory Factor analysis Fit Indices

Indices	Abbreviation	Recommended Criteria	Social Networking Impacts	Social Networking Addiction	Mental Health
Reliability test	Cronbach's Alpha	>7 good fit	-	0.926	-
Normed Chi-square	χ^2 / df	$1 < \chi^2 / df < 3$	2.65	2.954	2.424
Goodness-of-fit index	GFI	>0.80	0.814	0.952	0.835
Adjusted GFI	AGFI	>0.80	0.877	0.904	0.852
Normed fit index	NFI	>0.90	0.901	0.928	0.912
Comparative fit index	CFI	>0.95	0.957	0.934	0.951
Tucker–Lewis index	TLI	0 < TLI < 1	0.741	0.901	0.883
Root mean square error of approximation	RMSEA	<0.05 good fit < 0.08 acceptable fit	0.072	0.079	0.069

Source: Primary data

The confirmatory factor analysis fit indices and estimate table on social networking impacts, addiction and mental health indicates an acceptable model fit; this confirms that the measured variables represent the constructs for the sample data very well.

3.16 STATISTICAL TOOLS AND SOFTWARE PACKAGES

The 840 data obtained was subjected to quantitative statistical analyses using SPSS 22 and AMOS 24. Frequency analysis, Mean and Standard Deviation (SD) was done as part of Descriptive Statistics. Evaluation of the socio demographic profile was done through frequency analysis, t-test and anova. In the present study, the purpose of t-test was primarily to evaluate significant difference in mental health and social networking addiction on the basis of gender, place of residence and age at which they came to know about social networking. One-way ANOVA was done to evaluate the difference between socio demographic variables and mental health, social networking addiction. Mean analysis was done for reasons of social networking. Pearson product moment correlation was done to find out the relationship between study variables. In order to predict the influence of social networking impacts on addiction and mental health, regression analysis was conducted. The most influential impact of social networking was found out through confirmatory factor analysis. The relationship between social networking impacts, social networking addiction and mental health was explored through structural equation modeling. The data obtained through the semi-structured in-depth interview was transcribed appropriately and was then subjected to Thematic Analysis.

3.17 SUMMARY

This section of the thesis dealt with the research design of the study, overview of the research process, phases of research, period of study, sampling frame, variables, operational definitions, pilot study, process of scale development and the data collection method. The procedure for data collection, both quantitative as well as qualitative, was also discussed. The next chapter will focus on data analysis and interpretation of data.

CHAPTER 4

DATA ANALYSIS AND RESULTS

4.1 INTRODUCTION

The current study examined the influence of social networking on mental health, this chapter contains data analysis used to achieve significant findings to hold up the conceptual framework. Comprehensive analysis was done using the software packages SPSS 21, AMOS 24 and NVIVO 12. Frequency analysis, mean analysis, T test, anova, correlation, multiple regression and confirmatory factor analysis was done to test the statistical hypothesis.

Frequency analysis was done for the socio demographic profile, social networking addiction and mental health. Mean analysis was done for reasons for social networking. One way anova and T test was done to assess the difference in socio demographic profile on social networking addiction and mental health. In order to explore the relationship between reasons for social networking and impacts of social networking on social networking addiction and mental health, Pearson product moment correlation analysis was done. Multiple regression was performed to evaluate the influence of social networking impacts on mental health, social networking addiction. The most influential impact of social networking on mental health was identified through confirmatory factor analysis. Structural equation modelling was performed to evaluate the fitness of the model. The influence of social networking on mental health was explored further through qualitative analysis.

4.2 SOCIO DEMOGRAPHIC PROFILE

The basic information related to age, school, gender, religion, place of residence, living place, the person who is staying with the adolescent (with whom staying), type of family, current relationship status of parents, number of best friends and history of illness in the family was identified to understand the demographic background.

Table 4.1 Demographic Profile of the Adolescents

Demographic Variables		Frequency	Percentage
Age	15 Years	280	33.33%
	16 Years	280	33.33%
	17 Years	280	33.34%
School	Government	280	33.33%
	Aided	280	33.33%
	Unaided	280	33.34%
Gender	Male	420	50.00%
	Female	420	50.00%
Religion	Hindu	449	53.45%
	Muslim	59	7.02%
	Christian	326	38.82%
	Atheist	6	0.71%
Place of Residence	Urban	466	55.48%
	Rural	374	44.52%
Living Place	Own House	645	76.79%
	Hostel	126	15.00%
	Paying Guest	69	8.21%
The Person Who is Staying with the Adolescent (with Whom Staying)	Parents	681	81.07%
	Relatives	26	3.10%
	Friends	133	15.83%
Type of Family	Nuclear	685	81.55%
	Joint	132	15.71%
	Extended	23	2.74%
Current Relationship Status of Parents	Widowed	57	6.79%
	Divorced	10	1.19%
	Separated	26	3.10%
	Living With Spouse	696	82.86%
	Others	51	6.06%
Number of Best Friends	< 3	238	28.33%
	>3	556	66.19%
	Nil	46	5.48%
History of Illness in the Family	Mental Illness	152	18.10%
	Physical Illness	688	81.90%
	Drug Abuse	0	0.00%

Source: Primary data

Table 4.1 shows the demographic information of adolescents participated for the study on "influence of social networking on mental health among adolescents". The adolescents belongs to the age group 15-17 years; equal number of participants from each age group 280 (33.3%). From government, aided and unaided schools, 280 (33.3%) students participated in the study. 420 (50%) were males and 420 (50%) were female students. 449 (53.45%) were hindus, 59 (7.02%) were muslims, 326 (38.8%) were christians and 6 (0.71%) were atheist. 466 (55.48%) adolescents were from urban area and 374 (44.5%) belongs to rural area. 645 (76.8%) adolescents were staying in their own house, 126 (15%) were hostlers and 69 (8.3%) were staying as paying guest. 681 (81.1%) were staying with parents, 26 (3.1%) were staying with relatives and 133 (15.8%) of the adolescents were staying with their friends. 685 (81.5%) belongs to nuclear family whereas 132 (15.7%) belongs to joint family and 23 (2.7%) were from extended family. Among the adolescents, 57 (6.8%) were having only others with them, 10 (1.2%) of their mothers were divorcees, 26 (3.1%) of the adolescents parents were separated, 66 (82.8%) were living with both parents and 51 (6.1%) of the adolescents parents were having extra marital relationship. 556 (66.2%) were having more than three friends whereas 238 (28.4%) were having less than three friends. 46 (5.5%) were with no friends. Physical illness 688 (81.9%) was more prevalent in the adolescents family than mental illness152 (18.1%).

Table 4.2 Demographic Profile of the Parents

Parents Information		Frequency	Percentage
Education Status of Mother	Profession or Honours	51	6.07%
	Graduate	148	17.62%
	Intermediate or Diploma	179	21.31%
	High School Certificate	333	39.64%
	Middle School Certificate	76	9.05%
	Primary School Certificate	42	5.00%
	Illiterate	11	1.31%
Education Status of Father	Profession or Honours	47	5.60%
	Graduate	103	12.26%
	Intermediate or Diploma	154	18.33%
	High School Certificate	400	47.61%
	Middle School Certificate	72	8.57%
	Primary School Certificate	36	4.29%
	Illiterate	28	3.33%
Occupation Status of Mother	Legislator, Senior Official, Manager	11	1.31%
	Professional	93	11.07%
	Technician, Associate Professional	15	1.79%
	Clerk	27	3.21%
	Skilled Worker, Shop & Market Sales Worker	78	9.29%
	Skilled Agricultural & Fishery Worker	27	3.21%
	Craft & Related Trade Worker	15	1.79%
	Plant & Machine Operator, Assemblers	3	0.36%
	Elementary Occupation	36	4.28%
	Unemployed	535	63.69%
Occupation Status of Father	Legislator, Senior Official, Manager	27	3.21%
	Professional	86	10.24%
	Technician, Associate Professional	42	5.00%
	Clerk	35	4.17%
	Skilled Worker, Shop &Market Sales Worker	206	24.52%
	Skilled Agricultural & Fishery Worker	218	25.95%
	Craft & Related Trade Worker	19	2.26%
	Plant & Machine Operator, Assemblers	17	2.02%
	Elementary Occupation	134	15.95%
	Unemployed	56	6.68%
Income	Above Rupees 78,063	36	4.29%
	Rupees 39033 To 78062	88	10.48%
	Rupees 29200 To 39032	80	9.52%
	Rupees19516 To 29199	83	9.88%
	Rupees 11708 To 19515	116	13.81%
	Rupees 3908 To 11707	228	27.14%
	Less Than Rupees 3907	209	24.88%

Source: Primary data

Above Table 4.2 shows the parents information of the adolescents in this study. 51 (6.1%) of the mothers and 47 (5.7%) of the adolescents fathers have done Honors, 148 (17.6%) of the adolescents mothers and 103 (12.2%) of the fathers were Graduates, 179 (21.3%) of the mothers and 154 (18.3%) of the fathers has done Intermediate Or Diploma, 333 (39.6%) of the mothers and 400 (47.6%) of the fathers has done High School Certificate, 76 (9.1%) of the mothers and 72 (8.5%) of the fathers educated till Middle School Certificate, 42 (5%) of the mothers and 36 (4.2%) of the fathers has studied Primary School Certificate and 11 (1.3%) of the mothers and 28 (3.3%) of the fathers were Illiterate. 11 (1.3%) of the mothers and 27 (3.2%) of the fathers were Legislator / Senior Official / Manager whereas 93 (11.1%) of the mothers and 86 (10.2%) of the fathers were Professional. 15 (1.7%) of the mothers and 42 (5%) of the fathers were Technician / Associate Professional. 27 (3.2%) of the mothers and 35 (4.1%) of the fathers were doing clerical job.

78(9.2%) of the mothers and 206(24.5%) of the fathers were belonging to Skilled Worker, Shop & Market Sales Worker, 27(3.2%) of the mothers and 218 (25.9%) of the fathers were Skilled Agricultural & Fishery Worker. 15 (1.7) of the mothers and 19 (2.2%) of the fathers were Craft & Related Trade Worker. 3 (0.3%) of the mothers and 17 (2.1%) of the fathers were doing Plant & Machine Operator job, Assemblers. 36 (4.2%) of the mothers and 134 (15.9%) of the fathers were doing Elementary Occupation. Out of the 840 adolescents, 535 (63.6%) of mothers and 56 (6.6%) of the fathers were Unemployed.

With respect to the family income, 36 (4.2%) of them were having an income above Rs.78,063,88 (10.4%) between 39033-78062, 80 (9.5%) between 29200-39032, 83 (9.8%) between 19516-29199, 116 (13.8%) between 11708-19515, 228 (27.1%) between 3908-11707 and 209 (24.8%) were having an income of less than 3907.

4.3 EXTENT OF SOCIAL NETWORKING AND MENTAL HEALTH

Table 4.3 Social Networking Addiction and Mental Health

Social Networking Addiction and Mental Health		Number	Percentage
Social Networking Addiction	No Addiction	536	63.81%
	Mild	243	28.92%
	Moderate	47	5.60%
	Severe	14	1.67%
Mental Health	Low Mental Health	453	53.93%
	High Mental Health	387	46.07%

Source: Primary data

The above Table 4.3, reveals that 63.8% of the adolescents (n=536) engage in social networking without any addiction; whereas 28.9% (n=243) were addicted mildly; 5.6% (n=47) moderately and only 1.7% (n=14) were severely addicted. Among them 53.9% (n=453) were found to have low mental health and 46.1% (n=387) were having high mental health.

4.4 MEAN ANALYSIS

Table 4.4 Mean Analysis of Reasons for Social Networking

Sl No.	Item	Maximum Score	Mean Sore	SD	% of Mean Score
	Reason For Preferring Social Networking:				
1	Low Cost-Affordability	5	2.47	1.04	49.40%
2	Easy Accessibility-Accessibility	5	1.92	0.79	38.40%
3	Privacy-Anonymity	5	2.56	1.12	51.20%
4	Satisfaction of Need-Approximation	5	2.26	1.02	45.20%
5	Curiosity-Ambiguity	5	2.22	1.04	44.40%
6	Worldwide Acceptance-Acceptability	5	1.93	1.02	38.60%
7	Thinking that it is a Part of Life-Accommodation	5	2.85	1.25	57.00%
8	Freedom–Autonomy	5	2.54	1.18	50.80%
9	Feeling that Everything is Available in Internet-Availability	5	2.30	1.18	46.00%
10	Increased Interest in using Smart Phone	5	2.40	1.12	48.00%

Sl No.	Item	Maximum Score	Mean Sore	SD	% Of Mean Score
11	Less Monitoring of Parents	5	3.41	1.16	68.20%
12	Poor Parent-Child Relationship	5	3.48	1.30	69.60%
13	Influence of Friends	5	2.60	1.12	52.00%
14	Escaping from Studies	5	3.27	1.30	65.40%
15	Opportunity to Forget Previous Bad Experience	5	2.89	1.26	57.80%
16	Lack of Interest in Hobbies	5	3.14	1.23	62.80%
17	Lack of Life Satisfaction	5	3.35	1.18	67.00%
18	Reducing Suicidal Thoughts	5	3.36	1.37	67.20%
19	Fear on Face to Face Interaction	5	3.51	1.17	70.20%
20	Reducing Stress	5	2.41	1.19	48.20%
21	Reducing Nervousness	5	2.74	1.21	54.80%
22	Excessive Web Surfing	5	2.47	1.04	49.40%
23	Interest in Sending Threatening Email, to Frighten Others	5	1.92	0.79	38.40%
24	Increased Interest in Online Sex	5	2.56	1.12	51.20%
	Reason for Social Networking Habit:				
1	I use it Regularly	5	3.13	1.21	62.60%
2	I Think it is Time-Consuming	5	3.68	1.21	73.60%
3	I Feel Anxious, When the Network is not Available	5	3.95	1.18	79.00%
4	I Repeatedly Check Phone for Messages	5	2.38	1.27	47.60%
5	I Like Social Networking, Because of Constant Availability	5	2.24	1.23	44.80%
6	I Prefer Mobile Chat Over Face to Face Communication	5	2.58	1.34	51.60%
7	I Feel there is Fear of Missing out	5	2.53	1.31	50.60%
8	I can Form my Identity	5	1.98	1.27	39.60%
9	I get Social Support	5	1.79	1.12	35.80%
	Reasons for Engaging in Social Networking(Purpose):				
1	To Interact with Others	5	3.06	1.30	61.20%
2	To Establish and Maintain Relationship with Others	5	3.04	1.34	60.80%
3	To Increase the Knowledge Level	5	3.32	1.34	66.40%
4	To have Entertainment	5	3.51	1.29	70.20%
5	To Purchase Things Online	5	2.75	1.36	55.00%

Source: Primary data

Out of the 840 adolescents, the mean value of reasons of social networking was noted highest in fear on face to face interaction -3.51 with the corresponding standard deviation 1.17; whereas the lowest mean was for Accessibility and 'Interest in Sending Threatening Email, to Frighten Others' -1.92 with standard deviation 0.79. Reasons for social networking habit mean value was more for "I feel anxious, when the network is not available" -3.95 with the corresponding standard deviation, while the mean value was lowest for 1.18. While concerned to the purpose of social networking, the mean value was highest for entertainment 3.51 with the corresponding standard deviation 1.29 and lowest for online purchasing -2.75 with standard deviation 1.36.

4.5 ANOVA - SOCIO DEMOGRAPHIC PROFILE

4.5.1 Difference in Mental Health, Social Networking Addiction in Terms of Age

H5: There is significant difference in mental health in terms of age.

H6: There is significant difference in social networking addiction in terms of age.

Table 4.5 One-Way Anova- Difference in Mental Health, Social Networking Addiction in Terms of Age

Variables	Groups	Sum of squares	Df	Mean square	F	Sig.
Mental Health	Between groups	4756.588	2	2378.294	13.40	0.001***
	Within groups	148579.693	837	177.515		
	Total	**153336.281**	**839**			
Social networking addiction	Between groups	27.117	2	13.558	0.46	0.63#
	Within groups	24707.664	837	29.519		
	Total	**24734.781**	**839**			

Source: Primary data
*** indicates significance at 0.001 levels # indicates no significance at 0.05 levels

According to the Table 4.5 there exists the presence of significant difference in mental health, but there exists no significant difference in social networking addiction in terms of age among the adolescents. Thus, H5: There is significant difference in mental health in terms of age is accepted whereas; H6: There is significant difference in social networking addiction in terms of age was rejected.

Table 4.6 Duncan Test-Difference in Mental Health in Terms of Age

Age	N	Subset of alpha = 0.05*	
		1	2
16	280	45.92	
17	280	48.03	
15	280		51.68
Sig.		0.061	1.000

Source: Primary data
*Mean values appearing in the same subset are not significantly different from each other

Duncan test was done to explore the exact difference, results from the above Table 4.6 reveals that people of age 15 are having better mental health when compared to those of age 16 and 17.

4.5.2 Difference in Mental Health, Social Networking Addiction in terms of Gender

H7: There is significant difference in mental health in terms of gender.

H8: There is significant difference in social networking addiction in terms of gender.

Table 4.7 T test - Difference in Mental Health, Social Networking Addiction in terms of Gender

Variables	Sample	N	Mean	S. D	t- value	Sig.
Mental Health	Male	420	48.57	13.94	0.06	0.95#
	Female	420	48.52	13.10		
	Total	**840**	**48.55**	**13.52**		
Social Networking Addiction	Male	420	13.00	5.57	0.33	0.74#
	Female	420	12.88	5.29		
	Total	**840**	**12.94**	**5.43**		

Source: Primary data
# indicates no significance at 0.05 levels

Table 4.7 shows no significant difference in mental health and social networking addiction in terms of gender. Hence, hypothesis H7: There is significant difference in mental health in terms of gender and H8: There is significant difference in social networking addiction in terms of gender was rejected.

4.5.3 Difference in Mental Health and Social Networking Addiction in terms of Religion

H9: There is significant difference in mental health in terms of religion.

H10: There is significant difference in social networking addiction in terms of religion.

Table 4.8 One-Way ANOVA - Difference in Mental Health and Social Networking Addiction in terms of Religion

Variables	Groups	Sum of squares	Df	Mean square	F	Sig.
Mental Health	Between groups	6611.501	3	2203.83	12.56	0.001***
	Within groups	146724.780	836	175.51		
	Total	**153336.281**	**839**			
Social networking addiction	Between groups	115.194	3	38.40	1.30	0.27#
	Within groups	24619.587	836	29.45		
	Total	**24734.781**	**839**			

Source: Primary data
Note: *** indicates significance at 0.001 levels
# indicates no significance at 0.05 levels

The results from the above Table 4.8, indicate significant difference in mental health, but no significant difference was observed in social networking addiction in terms of religion. Hence the hypotheses, H9: There is significant difference in mental health in terms of religion is accepted while, H10: There is significant difference in social networking addiction in terms of religion is rejected.

Table 4.9 Duncan Test - Difference in Mental Health in terms of Religion

Religion	N	Subset for alpha = 0.05	
		1	2
Atheist	6	34.17	
Hindu	449		46.36
Muslim	59		49.42
Christian	326		51.67
Sig.		1.000	0.221

Source: Primary data
*Mean values appearing in the same subset are not significantly different from each other

Duncan test was done to further assess the difference exactly, above Duncan test Table 4.9 reveals that atheists have low mental health when compared to the adolescents of other religion.

4.5.4 Difference in Mental Health and social Networking Addiction in terms of Place of Residence

H11: There is significant difference in mental health in terms of place of residence.

H12: There is significant difference in social networking addiction in terms of place of residence.

Table 4.10 T test - Difference in Mental Health and Social Networking Addiction in terms of Place of Residence

Variables	Sample	N	Mean	S. D	t-value	Sig.
Mental Health	Urban	420	49.03	13.55	1.15	0.25#
	Rural	420	47.95	13.48		
	Total	**840**	**48.55**	**13.52**		
Social Networking Addiction	Urban	420	12.91	5.35	0.19	0.85#
	Rural	420	12.98	5.54		
	Total	**840**	**12.94**	**5.43**		

Source: Primary data
# indicates no significance at 0.05 levels

The findings of independent sample t-test disclose that there exists no significant difference in mental health and social networking addiction among adolescents in terms of their place of residence. Therefore, both H11: There is significant difference in mental health in terms of place of residence and H12: There is significant difference in social networking addiction in terms of place of residence is rejected.

4.5.5 Difference in Mental Health and Social Networking Addiction in terms of Living Place

H13: There is significant difference in mental health in terms of living place.

H14: There is significant difference in social networking addiction in terms of living place.

Table 4.11 One-Way ANOVA - Difference in Mental Health and Social Networking Addiction in terms of Living Place

Variables	Groups	Sum of squares	Df	Mean square	F	Sig.
Mental Health	Between groups	205.896	2	102.948	0.56	0.57#
	Within groups	153130.385	837	182.951		
	Total	**153336.281**	**839**			
Social networking addiction	Between groups	1.444	2	.722	0.02	0.98#
	Within groups	24733.337	837	29.550		
	Total	**24734.781**	**839**			

Source: Primary data
Note: # indicates no significance at 0.01 levels

Above Table 4.11 projects that there exists no significant difference in mental health and social networking addiction among adolescents on the basis of living place. For this reason both the hypothesis H13: There is significant difference in mental health in terms of living place and H14: There is significant difference in social networking addiction in terms of living place is rejected.

4.5.6 Difference in Mental Health and Social Networking Addiction in terms of With Whom Staying

H15: There is significant difference in mental health in terms of with whom staying.

H16: There is significant difference in social networking addiction in terms of with whom staying

Table 4.12 One-Way ANOVA- Difference in Mental Health and Social Networking Addiction in terms of With Whom Staying

Variables	Groups	Sum of squares	DF	Mean square	F	Sig.
Mental Health	Between groups	23.190	2	11.595	0.06	0.94#
	Within groups	153313.091	837	183.170		
	Total	153336.281	839			
Social networking addiction	Between groups	6.055	2	3.027	0.10	0.90#
	Within groups	24728.726	837	29.544		
	Total	24734.781	839			

Source: Primary data
Note: # indicates no significance at 0.05 levels

As publicized in Table 4.12 there is no significant difference in mental health and social networking addiction in terms of with whom staying. That is why H15: There is significant difference in mental health in terms of with whom staying and H16: There is significant difference in social networking addiction in terms of with whom staying is rejected.

4.5.7 Difference in Mental Health and Social Networking Addiction in terms of Type of Family

H17: There is significant difference in mental health in terms of type of family.

H18: There is significant difference in social networking addiction in terms of type of family

Table 4.13 One-Way ANOVA Difference in Mental Health and Social Networking Addiction in terms of Type of Family

Variables	Groups	Sum of squares	Df	Mean square	F	Sig.
Mental Health	Between groups	209.090	2	104.545	0.57	0.57#
	Within groups	153127.191	837	182.948		
	Total	**153336.281**	**839**			
Social networking addiction	Between groups	29.645	2	14.822	0.50	0.61#
	Within groups	24705.136	837	29.516		
	Total	**24734.781**	**839**			

Source: Primary data
Note: # indicates no significance at 0.05 levels

The results of Table 4.13 a specify no significant difference in mental health and social networking addiction in terms of type of family. Thus H17: There is significant difference in mental health in terms of type of family and H18: There is significant difference in social networking addiction in terms of type of family is rejected.

4.5.8 Difference in Mental Health and Social Networking Addiction in terms of Current Relationship Status of Parents

H19: There is significant difference in mental health in terms of current relationship status of parents.

H20: There is significant difference in social networking addiction in terms of current relationship status of parents.

Table 4.14 One-Way ANOVA Difference in Mental Health and Social Networking Addiction in Terms of Current Relationship Status of Parents

Variables	Groups	Sum of squares	Df	Mean square	F	Sig.
Mental Health	Between groups	703.637	4	175.91	0.96	0.43#
	Within groups	152632.644	835	182.79		
	Total	**153336.281**	**837**			
Social networking addiction	Between groups	66.282	4	16.57	0.56	0.69#
	Within groups	24668.499	835	29.54		
	Total	**24734.781**	**837**			

Source: Primary data
Note: # indicates no significance at 0.05levels

Above Table 4.14 denotes no significant difference in mental health and social networking addiction - in terms of current relationship status of parents. Hence both the hypothesis H19: There is significant difference in mental health in terms of current relationship status of parents and H20: There is significant difference in social networking addiction in terms of current relationship status of parents is rejected.

4.5.9 Difference in Mental Health and Social Networking Addiction in terms of Number of Best Friends

H21: There is significant difference in mental health in terms of number of best friends.

H22: There is significant difference in social networking addiction in terms of number of best friends

Table 4.15 One-Way ANOVA-Difference in Mental Health and Social Networking Addiction in terms of Number of Friends

Variables	Groups	Sum of squares	Df	Mean square	F	Sig.
Mental Health	Between groups	1210.959	5	242.192	3.39	0.25#
	Within groups	152125.322	834	182.404		
	Total	**153336.281**	**839**			
Social networking addiction	Between groups	211.808	5	42.362	3.32	0.05*
	Within groups	24522.973	834	29.404		
	Total	**24734.781**	**839**			

Source: Primary data
*** indicates significance at 0.05 levels   # indicates no significance at 0.05 levels

According to Table 4.15 there exists the presence of no significant difference in mental health, but there exists significant difference in social networking addiction in terms of number of best friends. Thus, hypothesis H21: There is significant difference in mental health in terms of number of best friends is rejected whereas H22: There is significant difference in social networking addiction in terms of number of best friends is accepted.

Table 4.16 Duncan Test - Difference in Social Networking Addiction in terms of Number of Friends

Best friends	N	Subset for alpha = 0.05	
		1	2
0	46	10.96	
1	56		12.63
2	74		12.82
3	81		12.91
4	475		13.13
5	108		13.19
Sig.		0.055	0.569

Source: Primary data
Means for groups in homogeneous subsets are displayed.

Duncan test was done to explore the difference, Table 4.16 shows that addiction is less among adolescents with no friends than with friends.

4.5.10 Difference in Mental Health and Social Networking Addiction in terms of Type of School

H23: There is significant difference in mental health in terms of type of school.

H24: There is significant difference in social networking addiction in terms of type of school.

Table 4.17 One-Way ANOVA Difference in Mental Health and Social Networking Addiction in terms of Type of School

Variables	Groups	Sum of squares	Df	Mean square	F	Sig.
Mental Health	Between groups	507.317	2	253.658	1.39	0.20#
	Within groups	152828.964	837	182.591		
	Total	**153336.281**	**839**			
Social networking addiction	Between groups	3.031	2	1.515	0.05	0.95#
	Within groups	24731.750	837	29.548		
	Total	**24734.781**	**839**			

Source: Primary data
# indicates no significance at 0.05levels

The Table 4.17 clearly shows no significant difference in mental health and social networking addiction among the adolescents in terms of the type of school they are studying. Hence both the hypothesis H23: There is significant difference in mental health in terms of type of school and H24: There is significant difference in social networking addiction in terms of type of school is rejected.

4.5.11 Difference in Mental Health and Social Networking Addiction in terms of History of Illness in the Family

H25: There is significant difference in mental health in terms of history of illness in the family.

H26: There is significant difference in social networking addiction in terms of history of illness in the family.

Table 4.18 T Test - Difference in Mental Health and Social Networking Addiction in terms of History of Illness in the Family

Variables	Groups	N	Mean	S. D	t-value	Sig.
Mental Health	Physical illness	688	48.32	13.66	1.09	0.30#
	Mental illness	152	49.58	12.86		
	Total	**840**	**48.55**	**13.52**		
Social Networking Addiction	Physical illness	688	13.11	5.50	4.04	0.05*
	Mental illness	152	12.14	5.06		
	Total	**840**	**12.94**	**5.43**		

Source: Primary data

*** indicates significance at 0.05 levels # indicates no significance at 0.05 levels

According to Table 4.18, there exists the presence of no significant difference in mental health, but there exists significant difference in social networking addiction among the adolescents in terms of history of illness. Thus, hypothesis H25: There is significant difference in mental health in terms of history of illness in the family is rejected; while H26: There is significant difference in social networking addiction in terms of history of illness in the family is accepted.

4.5.12 Difference in Mental Health and Social Networking Addiction in terms of Education Status of Mother

H27: There is significant difference in mental health in terms of education status of mother.

H28: There is significant difference in social networking addiction in terms of education status of mother.

Table 4.19 One-Way ANOVA Difference in Mental Health and Social Networking Addiction in terms of Education Status of Mother

Variables	Groups	Sum of squares	Df	Mean square	F	Sig.
Mental Health	Between groups	338.19	6	56.37	0.31	0.93#
	Within groups	152998.09	833	183.67		
	Total	**153336.28**	**839**			
Social networking addiction	Between groups	338.31	6	56.39	1.93	0.07#
	Within groups	24396.47	833	29.29		
	Total	**24734.78**	**839**			

Source: Primary data
# indicates no significance at 0.05level

The Table 4.19 clearly shows no significant difference in mental health and social networking addiction among the adolescents in terms of the education status of mother. Hence hypothesis H27: There is significant difference in mental health in terms of education status of mother and H28: There is significant difference in social networking addiction in terms of education status of mother is rejected.

4.5.13 Difference in Mental Health and Social Networking Addiction in terms of Education Status of Father

H29: There is significant difference in mental health in terms of education status of father.

H30: There is significant difference in social networking addiction in terms of education status of father.

Table 4.20 One-Way ANOVA Difference in Mental Health and Social Networking Addiction in terms of Education Status of Father

Variables	Groups	Sum of squares	Df	Mean square	F	Sig.
Mental Health	Between groups	758.42	6	126.40	0.69	0.66#
	Within groups	152577.86	833	183.17		
	Total	**153336.28**	**839**			
Social networking addiction	Between groups	356.23	6	59.37	2.03	0.06#
	Within groups	24378.55	833	29.27		
	Total	**24734.78**	**839**			

Source: Primary data
# indicates no significance at 0.05level

The Tables 4.20 clearly shows no significant difference in mental health and social networking addiction among the adolescents in terms of education status of father. Hence hypothesis H29: There is significant difference in mental health in terms of education status of father and H30: There is significant difference in social networking addiction in terms of education status of father is rejected.

4.5.14 Difference in Mental Health and Social Networking Addiction in terms of Occupation Status of Mother

H31: There is significant difference in mental health in terms of occupation status of mother.

H32: There is significant difference in social networking addiction in terms of occupation status of mother.

Table 4.21 One-Way ANOVA-Difference in Mental Health and Social Networking Addiction in terms of Occupation Status of Mother

Variables	Groups	Sum of squares	Df	Mean square	F	Sig.
Mental Health	Between groups	758.42	9	126.40	1.54	0.13#
	Within groups	152577.86	833	183.17		
	Total	**153336.28**	**842**			
Social networking addiction	Between groups	356.23	9	59.37	2.57	0.01**
	Within groups	24378.55	833	29.27		
	Total	**24734.78**	**842**			

Source: Primary data
** indicates significance at 0.01 levels # indicates no significance at 0.05 levels

According to Table 4.21, there exists no significant difference in mental health, but there exists significant difference in social networking addiction in terms of occupation status of mother. Thus, hypothesis number H31: There is significant difference in mental health in terms of occupation status of mother is rejected whereas; H32: There is significant difference in social networking addiction in terms of occupation status of mother is accepted.

Table 4.22 Duncan Test - Difference in Social Networking Addiction in terms of Occupation Status of Mother

Occupation Status of Mother	N	Subset for alpha = 0.05	
		1	2
Plant & Machine Operator, Assemblers	3	11.00	
Skilled Agricultural & Fishery Worker	27	11.33	
Elementary Occupation	36	12.08	
Professional	93	12.44	
Unemployed	535	12.81	
Technician, Associate Professional	15	13.40	
Clerk	27	13.52	
Legislator, Senior Official, Manager	11	13.55	
Skilled Worker, Shop & Market, Sales Worker	78	14.01	
Craft & Related Trade Worker	15		18.27
Sig.		0.211	1.000

Source: Primary data
Means for groups in homogeneous subsets are displayed.

From the above Duncan Table 4.22, it is clear that the adolescents with mother's occupation as skilled workers, shops, markets, sales worker craft and related trade worker were having difference in addiction (high) when compared to others.

4.5.15 Difference in Mental Health and Social Networking Addiction in terms of Occupation Status of Father

H33: There is significant difference in mental health in terms of occupation status of father.

H34: There is significant difference in social networking addiction in terms of occupation status of father.

Table 4.23 One-Way ANOVA - Difference in Mental Health and Social Networking Addiction in terms of Occupation Status of Father

Variables	Groups	Sum of squares	Df	Mean square	F	Sig.
Mental Health	Between groups	2111.58	9	234.62	1.28	0.24#
	Within groups	151224.69	830	182.29		
	Total	**153336.27**	**839**			
Social networking addiction	Between groups	597.24	9	66.360	2.28	0.05*
	Within groups	24137.54	830	29.08		
	Total	**24734.78**	**839**			

Source: Primary data
** indicates significance at 0.05 levels # indicates no significance at 0.05 levels

According to Tables 4.23, there exists the presence of no significant difference in mental health, but there exists significant difference in social networking addiction in terms of occupation status of father among the adolescents. Thus, hypothesis H33: There is significant difference in mental health in terms of occupation status of father is rejected, while H34: There is significant difference in social networking addiction in terms of occupation status of father is accepted.

Table 4.24 Duncan Test - Difference in Social Networking Addiction in terms of Occupation Status of Father

Occupation Status of Father	N	Subset for alpha = 0.05		
		1	2	3
Skilled Agricultural & Fishery Worker	218	12.33		
Elementary Occupation	134	12.35		
Unemployed	56	12.61	12.61	
Legislator, Senior Official, Manager	27	12.67	12.67	
Skilled Worker, Shop & Markets Sales worker	206	13.08	13.08	
Professional	86	13.16	13.16	
Clerk	35	13.26	13.26	
Plant & Machine Operator, Assemblers	17	14.18	14.18	14.18
Technician, Associate Professional	42		15.19	15.19
Craft & Related Trade Worker	19			16.26
Sig.		0.196	0.063	0.101

Source: Primary data
Means for groups in homogeneous subsets are displayed.

Duncan test explored the difference in social networking addiction among the different categories. Addiction was more noticed among adolescents whose fathers were trade and craft workers when compared with other workers as per the Duncan Table 4.24.

4.5.16 Difference in Mental Health and Social Networking Addiction in terms of Income

H35: There is significant difference in mental health in terms of income.

H36: There is significant difference in social networking addiction in terms of income

Table 4.25 One-Way ANOVA- Difference in Mental Health and Social Networking Addiction in terms of Income

Variables	Groups	Sum of squares	Df	Mean square	F	Sig.
Mental Health	Between groups	3064.19	6	510.7-	2.83	0.01**
	Within groups	150272.09	833	180.40		
	Total	**153336.28**	**839**			
Social networking addiction	Between groups	542.924	6	90.487	3.12	0.01**
	Within groups	24191.857	833	29.042		
	Total	**24734.781**	**839**			

Source: Primary data
** indicates significance at 0.01levels

According to Tables 4.25 there exists the presence of significant difference among adolescents in their mental health and social networking addiction in terms of income. Thus, both the hypothesis H35: There is significant difference in mental health in terms of income and H36: There is significant difference in social networking addiction in terms of income is accepted.

Table 4.26 Duncan Test – Difference in Mental Health in terms of Income

Income	N	Subset for alpha = 0.05		
		1	2	3
Rupees19516 to 29199	83	43.77		
Rupees 39033 to 78062	88	47.14	47.14	
Rupees 3908 to 11707	228		48.49	48.49
Rupees 29200 to 39032	80		48.71	48.71
Rupees 11708 to 19515	116		49.66	49.66
Less than Rupees 3907	209		49.74	49.74
Above Rupees 78,063	36			52.47
Sig.		0.101	0.266	0.084

Source: Primary data
Means for groups in homogeneous subsets are displayed.

Mental health was more among adolescents with high economic status than with low economic status as per the Duncan Table 4.26.

Table 4.27 Duncan Test – Difference in Mental Health and Social Networking Addiction in terms of Income

Income	N	Subset for alpha = 0.05		
		1	2	3
Above Rupees 78,063	36	11.56		
Less than Rupees 3907	209	12.02	12.02	
Rupees 11708 to 19515	116	12.74	12.74	12.74
Rupees 3908 to 11707	228	12.93	12.93	12.93
Rupees 39033 to 78062	88		13.75	13.75
Rupees 29200 to 39032	80			13.99
Rupees19516 to 29199	83			14.28
Sig.		0.130	0.054	0.097

Source: Primary data
Means for groups in homogeneous subsets are displayed.

Addiction was more noticed in adolescents with high economic status than with low economic status.

As per the Duncan Table 4.27, social networking addiction is more among the highest economic category adolescents than with others.

4.6 CORRELATION ANALYSIS

H37: There is significant relationship between reasons for social networking and addiction.

H38: There is significant relationship between reasons for social networking and mental health.

H39: There is significant relationship between social networking impacts and addiction.

H40: There is significant relationship between social networking impacts and mental health.

H41: There is significant relationship between social networking addiction and mental health.

Table 4.28 Correlation Analysis of Reasons for Social Networking, Social Networking Impacts on Social Networking Addiction, Mental Health

Variables		Mental health	Social Networking Addiction	Reason for preferring Social Networking	Reason for Social Networking Habit	Reason for Engaging in Social Networking	Physical impacts	Academic impacts	Psychological impacts	Adjustment impacts	Family impact
Mental health	Pearson Correlation	1	-.544**	-.328**	-.358**	-.377**	-.534**	-.510**	-.579**	-.547**	-.517**
	Sig. (2-tailed)		.000	.000	.000	.000	.000	.000	.000	.000	.000
	N		840	840	840	840	840	840	840	840	840
Social Networking Addiction	Pearson Correlation		1	.029	.511**	.295**	.563**	.502**	.509**	.481**	.488**
	Sig. (2-tailed)			.401	.000	.000	.000	.000	.000	.000	.000
	N			840	840	840	840	840	840	840	840
Reason for preferring Social Networking	Pearson Correlation			1	.186**	.286**	.201**	.233**	.206**	.358**	.273**
	Sig. (2-tailed)				.000	.000	.000	.000	.000	.000	.000
	N				840	840	840	840	840	840	840
Reason for Social Networking Habit	Pearson Correlation				1	.476**	.387**	.407**	.383**	.514**	.369**
	Sig. (2-tailed)					.000	.000	.000	.000	.000	.000
	N					840	840	840	840	840	840
Reason for Engaging in Social Networking	Pearson Correlation					1	.297**	.276**	.238**	.367**	.264**
	Sig. (2-tailed)						.000	.000	.000	.000	.000
	N						840	840	840	840	840
Physical impacts	Pearson Correlation						1	.536**	.546**	.606**	.606**
	Sig. (2-tailed)							.000	.000	.000	.000
	N							840	840	840	840
Academic impacts	Pearson Correlation							1	.716**	.633**	.620**
	Sig. (2-tailed)								.000	.000	.000
	N								840	840	840

Variables		Mental health	Social Networking Addiction	Reason for preferring Social Networking	Reason for Social Networking Habit	Reason for Engaging in Social Networking	Physical impacts	Academic impacts	Psychological impacts	Adjustment impacts	Family impact
Psycho-logical impacts	Pearson Correlation								1	.619**	.630**
	Sig. (2-tailed)									.000	.000
	N									840	840
Adjustment impacts	Pearson Correlation									1	.736**
	Sig. (2-tailed)										.000
	N										840
Family impact	Pearson Correlation										1
	Sig. (2-tailed)										
	N										
Depression	Pearson Correlation										
	Sig. (2-tailed)										
	N										
Anxiety	Pearson Correlation										
	Sig. (2-tailed)										
	N										

Source: Primary data
**. Correlation is significant at the 0.01 level (2-tailed).
*. Correlation is significant at the 0.05 level (2-tailed).

It is evident from Table 4.28 that there exists a significant positive correlation between reasons for preferring social networking (r=.029), reasons for social networking habit (r= .511**) and reasons for engaging in social networking (r= .295**) with addiction. This shows that as the intensity of social networking increases chances of getting addicted also increases. Thus hypotheses H37: There is significant relationship between reasons for social networking and addiction has been accepted.

From the Table 4.28, it is inferred that there exists a significant negative correlation between reasons for preferring social networking (r= -.328), reasons for social networking habit (r= -.358) and reasons for engaging in social networking (r= -.377) with mental health. Adolescents engage in social networking for various reasons, as the intensity of social networking increases mental health decreases. H38: There is significant relationship between reasons for social networking and mental health has been accepted.

It is also evident that there exists a significant positive correlation between social networking addiction and physical (r =.563**), academic (r =.502**), psychological (r = .509**) adjustment (r =.481**), and family impacts (r =.488**). This shows that when the impacts are more chances of addiction is also high. Hence hypotheses H39: There is significant relationship between social networking impacts and addiction has been accepted.

Adolescents, who engage in social networking excessively can have various impacts and will end up with low mental health. Mental health is related to physical (r = -.534**), academic (r = -.510**), psychological (r = -.579**), adjustment (r = -.547**), and family impacts (r = -.517**); there exists a negative relationship between them. As the social networking impacts increases, mental health reduces. Hence H40: There is significant relationship between social networking impacts and mental health has been accepted.

Negative relationship is observed between addiction (r = -.544**) and mental health. As addiction increases mental health deteriorates and hence, H41: There is significant relationship between social networking addiction and mental health is accepted.

4.7 MULTIPLE REGRESSION

Multiple regression analysis is done to check the influence of social networking impacts (independent variables) and addiction, mental health (dependent variables).

H42: There is significant influence of social networking impacts on addiction.

H43: There is significant influence of social networking impacts on mental health.

4.7.1 Multiple Regression - Influence of Social Networking Impacts on Social Networking Addiction

Table 4.29 Model Summary - Social Networking Impacts and Social Networking Addiction

Model	R	R Square	Adjusted R Square	Std. Error of the Estimate	Change Statistics				
					R Square Change	F Change	df1	df2	Sig. F Change
1	0.627[a]	0.393	0.389	4.381	0.393	107.959	5	834	0.000*

Source: Primary data * 1% level of significance

a. Dependent variable: Social Networking Addiction
b. Predictors (constant): Physical Impacts, Academic Impacts, Psychological Impacts, Adjustment Impacts and Familial Impacts

The Table 4.29 shows that the independent variables social networking impacts correlate 0.627 with the dependent variable addiction. The R square value gives goodness of fit measure and reflects the observed data clusters around the estimated regression line. In this study R square value is 0.393, which shows that only 39.3% of the variance is explained in this model. Even though the R square is moderate, significant coefficients is used to depict conclusion.

Table 4.30 ANOVA - Social Networking Impacts and Social Networking Addiction

Model		Sum of Squares	Df	Mean Square	F	Sig.
1	Regression	10358.197	5	2071.639	107.959	0.000*
	Residual	16003.684	834	19.189		
	Total	26361.881	839			

Source: Primary data * 1% level of significance

a. Dependent Variable: Social Networking Addiction
b. Predictors: (Constant): Physical Impacts, Academic Impacts, Psychological Impacts, Adjustment Impacts and Familial Impacts

ANOVA Table 4.30 shows that the significant value is less than 0.01, which means that the dependent variable social networking addiction is significantly predicted by the independent variables social networking impacts at 99 % of confidence level.

Table 4.31 Regression Coefficients - Social Networking Impacts and Social Networking Addiction

Model		Unstandardized Coefficients		Standardized Coefficients	T	Sig	Collinearity Statistics	
		B	Std. Error	Beta			Tolerance	VIF
1	(Constant)	4.562	0.403		11.319	0.000	3.771	5.353
	Physical Impacts	0.358	0.039	0.336	9.245	0.000	0.282	0.434
	Academic Impacts	0.241	0.070	0.144	3.438	0.001	0.103	0.378
	Psychological Impacts	0.169	0.046	0.155	3.710	0.000	0.080	0.258
	Adjustment Impacts	0.057	0.063	0.039	0.903	0.367	-0.067	0.181
	Familial Impacts	0.095	0.061	0.068	1.553	0.121	-0.025	0.215

Source: Primary data * 1% level of significance

The above Table 4.31 shows the coefficient values of the model. The p- value is significant ($p \leq 0.01$), at 1% level of significance for physical, academic and psychological impact. This shows that the independent variables physical, academic and psychological impact has a strong influence on social networking addiction.

Dependent variable= Constant + (B-Independent variables)

Social Networking Addiction = 4.562 + (0.358) Physical Impacts + (0.241) Academic Impacts + (0.169) Psychological + (0.057) Adjustment Impacts + (0.095) Familial Impacts.

From the results, while comparing the impacts, it is observed that the physical impact is found to be the most significant impact affecting the social networking addiction. As the social networking impacts increases, addiction also increases. Hence hypothesis H42: There is significant influence of social networking impacts on addiction is accepted.

4.7.2 Multiple Regression – Influence of Social Networking Impacts on Mental Health

Table 4.32 Model Summary - Social Networking Impacts and Mental Health

Model	R	R Square	Adjusted R Square	Std. Error of the Estimate	Change Statistics				
					R Square Change	F Change	df1	df2	Sig. F Change
1	0.653[a]	0.427	0.423	10.268	0.427	124.057	5	834	9.000*

Source: Primary data *1% level of significance

a. Dependent variable: Mental health.
b. Predictors (constant) Physical Impacts, Academic Impacts, Psychological Impacts, Adjustment Impacts and Familial Impacts.

Yue, (2004) suggested that R^2 value is used to determine, the extent of independent constructs facilitate to clarify the dependent construct, the R^2 value ranges from 0 to 1, as the value increases accuracy also increases. It is not easy to grant rules of thumb for satisfactory R^2 value as this depends on the model complexity and the research discipline (Hair et al 2013).

The above model summary Table 4.32 shows that the independent variables social networking impacts correlate 0.653 with the dependent variable mental health. The R square value gives goodness of fit measure and reflects the observed data clusters around the estimated regression line. In this study R square value is 0.427, which shows that only 42.7% of the variance is explained in this model. Even though the R square is moderate, significant coefficients will have used to draw conclusions.

Table 4.33 ANOVA - Social Networking Impacts and Mental Health

Model		Sum of Squares	Df	Mean Square	F	Sig.
1	Regression	65401.494	5	13080.299	124.057	0.000*
	Residual	87934.787	834	105.437		
	Total	153336.281	839			

Source: Primary data *1% level of significance

a. Dependent Variable: Mental health
b. Predictors: (Constant): Physical Impacts, Academic Impacts, Psychological Impacts, Adjustment Impacts and Familial Impacts

ANOVA Table 4.33 shows that the significant value is less than 0.01, which means that the dependent variable mental health is significantly predicted by the independent variable social networking impacts at 99 % of confidence level.

Table 4.34 Regression Coefficients for Social Networking Impacts and Mental Health

Model		Unstandardized Coefficients		Standardized Coefficients	T	Sig.	Collinearity Statistics	
		B	Std. Error	Beta			Tolerance	VIF
1	(Constant)	69.176	0.945		73.220	0.000		
	Physical Impacts	-0.559	0.091	-0.218	-6.165	0.000	0.550	1.819
	Academic Impacts	-0.201	0.164	-0.050	-1.225	0.221	0.416	2.406
	Psychological Impacts	-0.761	0.107	-0.290	-7.135	0.000	0.415	2.410
	Adjustment Impacts	-0.590	0.148	-0.169	-3.982	0.000	0.381	2.628
	Familial Impacts	-0.157	0.144	-0.046	-1.090	0.276	0.382	2.616

Source: Primary data * 1% level of significance

The above Table 4.34 shows the coefficient values of the model. The p-value is significant ($p \leq 0.01$), at 1% level of significance for physical, psychological and adjustment impact. This shows that the independent variables physical, psychological and adjustment impacts have a strong influence on mental health.

Dependent variable = Constant + (B-Independent variables)

Mental Health = 69.176+ (-0.559) Physical Impacts + (-0.201) Academic Impacts + (-0.761) Psychological Impacts + (-0.590) Adjustment Impacts + (-0.571) Familial Impacts.

From the results, while comparing the impacts, it is observed that the coefficient value of psychological impact is found to be the highest; the most significant impact affecting the mental health. Thus, it is clear that social networking impacts will reduce the mental health and therefore, H43: There is significant influence of social networking impacts on mental health is accepted.

4.8 STRUCTURAL EQUATION MODEL

Structural equation model is the graphical equivalent of its mathematical representation of a set of equations relating the dependent variables to their explanatory variables. These observed variables function as indicators of their respective underlying latent factors. Associated with each observed variable is an error terms which is associated with the factor being predicted. Errors associated with observed variables represent measurement error, which reflects on their adequacy in measuring the related underlying factors. Residual terms represent error in the prediction of endogenous factors from exogenous factors.

Certain symbols are used in path diagrams to denote hypothesized processes involving the entire system of variables. In particular, one-way arrows represent structural regression coefficients and thus indicating the impact of one variable on another. The observed variables of social networking impacts and mental health can be represented in the form of unidirectional arrows suggesting that these values are each influenced by their respective underlying factors. These path coefficients represent the magnitude of expected change in the observed variables for every change in the related latent variable. The one-way arrows pointing from the enclosed error terms in the improved measurement model indicate the impact of measurement error on the observed variables.

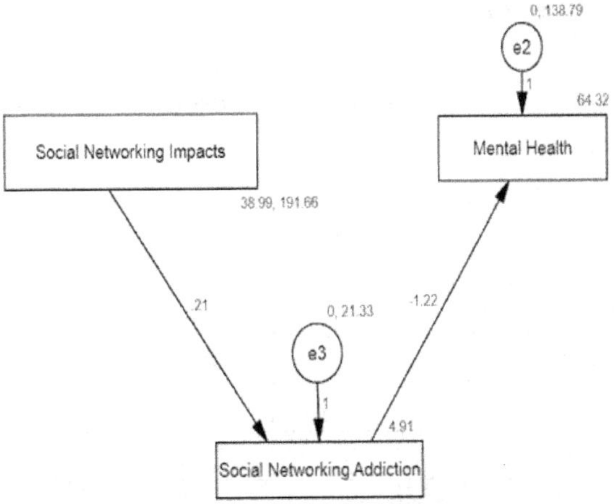

Figure 4.1 Structural Equation Model

In reviewing the model presented in Figure 4.1, it can be seen that there are unobserved latent factors and observed variables. This path analysis is an extension of the regression model. Path model diagram shows the independent, intermediate and dependent variables. A single-headed arrow shows the cause for the independent, intermediate and dependent variable. The one-way arrows pointing from the enclosed error terms in the improved measurement model indicate the impact of measurement error on the observed variables. In reviewing the path model, it can be seen that addiction is influenced by the impacts and mental health, which are the outcome of the present research. All the paths in the path model reflect the findings in the literature and the model shown in Figure 4.1 represents only the structural portion of the Structural Equation Model.

This model shows that social networking impact has a positive relation with social networking addiction and addiction has a negative relationship with mental health. Social networking addiction will in turn reduce the mental health of the addicted ones. Thus, from the model it is concluded that social networking impacts will lead to social networking addiction and addiction will lead to reduction in mental health. As the correlation and regression analysis go hand in hand, it gives a clear picture that this model is apt for this study.

4.8.1 Model Fitness

Table 4.35 Fit Statistics for the Model

Fit Statistic	Abbreviations	Bench Mark	Obtained
χ^2		-	5538.110
Degrees of Freedom	df	-	1004
χ^2 Significance		$P < 0.05$	0.935
χ^2 / df		< 5.0	0.5328
Goodness of Fit	GFI	> 0.90	0.989
Modified Goodness of Fit Index	AGFI	> 0.90	0.918
Normalized Fit Index	NFI	> 0.90	0.946
Comparative Fit Index	CFI	> 0.90	1.000
Incremental Fit Index	IFI	> 0.90	1.021
Tucker Lewis Index	TLI	> 0.90	1.321
Root Mean Square Error of Approximation	RMSEA	< 0.05	0.000
Root Mean Square Residual	RMR	< 0.05	0.0012
Standardized Root Mean Square Residual	SRMR	< 0.05	0.0258

Source: Primary data

A relatively small chi-square value supports the proposed theoretical model that is being tested. The AMOS output shows that for this model, the χ^2 value is 5538.110 which is small compared to the value of the independence model (12608.654). Hence, the theoretical model is supported. Even if the χ^2 is good, it is more appropriate to check the value of χ^2 divided by df (Wheaton, B., et al 1977). This is because the χ^2 statistic is very sensitive to the sample size and is no longer relied upon as a basis for acceptance or rejection (Vandenberg, R. J. 2006). Hence, chi-square (χ^2) divided by degrees of freedom is suggested as a metric for better-fit (Bentler, P. M., & Bonett, D. G. 1980), the ideal metric for a model with good fit does not exceed five. For the current model, χ^2 / df was 1.061 (χ^2 = 5538.110; df = 1004), suggesting the model is fit. The other different common model-fit measures shown in

Table 4.35 also suggests that the model is having overall goodness of fit. The confirmatory factor analysis showed an acceptable overall model fit and hence, the theorized model fits well with the observed data.

4.9 QUALITATIVE ANALYSIS

OBJECTVE: To explore the influence of social networking on mental health through qualitative analysis.

Inorder to further identify the adolescent's influence of social networking, an in-depth face to face interview was conducted with various research questions. The major themes and the subthemes identified are given in the Table 4.36.

Table 4.36 Thematic Analysis Out Put of Qualitative Analysis

Sl No.	Research Question	Major Themes	Sub Themes 1	Sub Themes 2
1	What is the purpose of social networking?	• Academics • Entertainment • Communication • Knowledge – insemination • Need satisfaction	• Learning • Fun – gaming • Resource sharing • Time pass • Social contact • Sexual satisfaction	Study presentation, doubt clearance, general knowledge, quiz, downloading and playing games, downloading / watching movies, songs, online sex, relaxation, chatting, sending messages, video call, downloading and reading books, watching news, online learning, preparing projects, sending photos / videos, interact with others.
2	What are the thoughts that emerge when engaged in social networking?	• Pleasant • Unpleasant • Constructive • Disruptive	• Encouraging thoughts • Discouraging thoughts • Thoughts related to communication • Thoughts related to sexuality	Think of meeting people, purchasing, need more time, use related thoughts, thoughts of using social media at inappropriate times, late night, sexual thoughts.

Sl No.	Research Question	Major Themes	Sub Themes 1	Sub Themes 2
3	What are the feelings (emotions) when engaged in social networking?	• Positive • Negative	• Enjoyment • Sadness • Anger • Happiness	Feel close and connected to people, feel safe and secure, sensory pleasure, get absorbed in activities, feel relaxed and at peace. Feel gloomy / frustrated when not able to connect to social media, irritated when someone interrupts the use. Feel related when involved in social networking. Happy, relief, refreshed, enjoyment, energetic, hopeful, thrilled, relaxed, comfortable, cheerfulness. Craziness, anger, irritation, "wow" feeling. Feel like killing when disrupted the use.
4	What are the impacts of social networking?	• Positive • Negative	• Physical, • Psychological • Social • Spiritual • Family • Adjustment	Relaxation, positivity, enhances mood, enhances creativity, academic achievement, increased performance, increased awareness, knowledge insemination, mingling with friends, time pass, increased knowledge, motivates, reduce heaviness of mind, encourages learning. Sleep / bodily issues, emotional issues, religious withdrawal, self-care neglect, interpersonal issue, headache, muscle pain, breathing difficulty, sleep issues, not interested in study / activities, feeling sad, anger, loss of interest in religious activities, quarrels, lying, spending money, change in daily routines and self-care, feel frustrated when not using it, family quarrels.

Sl No.	Research Question	Major Themes	Sub Themes 1	Sub Themes 2
5	What are the Perceived benefits of social networking?	• Increased knowledge • Psychological wellbeing	• Knowledge acquisition • Stress relief • Enjoyment	Reduced stress, gives fun, lots of information gain. Feel happy, feel satisfied, feel cherished, feels comfortable, reduces boredom / time pass, team spirit, diversion of negative thoughts, "we" feeling, privacy and independency. Online shopping. Can connect with / talk / chat / see even far way friends online without travelling, can see them at any time / whenever needed. Saves time, energy and money. Group interaction, clarification of doubts.
6	How social networking affects personal, academic and social life?	• Positively • Negatively • Encouraging • Discouraging	• Connectedness • Social interaction • Social isolation (social disconnectedness)	Meeting friends, keeping contact with friends.
7	Is social networking a healthy behavior?	• Beneficial	• Greater extent – beneficial • Need to be used with care	Proper use is beneficial, need in day today activities, helps in studies, gives regular updates, cannot be avoided.

Source: Primary data

From the qualitative analysis it was revealed that adolescents engage in social networking for entertainment, communication, knowledge insemination, online shopping and for need satisfaction. The thoughts and feelings that emerge in their mind include both pleasant and unpleasant one. Social networking has both positive and negative impacts, increased knowledge and psychological wellbeing was the benefits out of it. Social networking has positive effect in academic, social and personal life; healthy behavior as per the adolescents.

4.10 CONCLUSION

The study clearly answered the research questions and satisfied all the objectives which the researcher wanted to explore. Correlation analysis proved negative relationship between reasons, social networking impacts, addiction and mental health; whereas positive relationship between reasons, social networking impacts and social networking addiction. From the regression analysis also it is clear that as the social networking impacts increase, addiction increases and mental health reduces. Among the various impacts, psychological impact is proved to be the most influential impact. Structural equation model has confirmed model fit. Qualitative analysis also proved that if the intensity of social networking is increased, the adolescent can land up with impacts, addiction and thereby poor metal health.

CHAPTER 5

FINDINGS AND SUGGESTIONS

5.1 SOCIO DEMOGRAPHIC PROFILE OF THE ADOLESCENTS

5.1.1 Age, Religion and Income-Mental Health

The Anova finding proved that there exists significant difference among adolescents in their mental health in terms of age. Duncan test result revealed that 15 year old ones are mentally healthy when compared to those of age 16 and 17 years. Age is an important factor that contributes to many behavioral problems. Bhola & Mahakud (2014) stated that the age at which adolescents start social networking is 14.6 years; this can affect the mental health. There exists significant difference in mental health in terms of religion among the adolescents according to Anova test. Duncan test revealed that Atheists have low mental health whereas, Christians have high mental health. Religious beliefs help in increasing the physical and mental health. Behere et al (2018) reported that Christians have low rate of suicide; this shows that they are mentally healthy. Anova proved that there exists significant difference among adolescents in their mental health and addiction in terms of income. As per the Duncan test, mental health and addiction was more among the adolescents with high economic status than with low economic status. Study by Yu and Shek (2013) also showed that social networking addiction was less in low socio-economic class.

5.1.2 Demographic Profile of the Parents

5.1.2.1 Occupation Status of Parents - Social Networking

From the Anova test, it was found that there exists significant difference among adolescents in their social networking in terms of occupation status of parents. Duncan test revealed that adolescents with mother's occupation as skilled workers, shops, markets, sales workers, craft and related trade workers had difference in addiction (high) when compared to others, addiction was more noticed among adolescents whose fathers were trade and craft workers when compared with other workers. The study finding is in consistent with HASAN, M., & HALDER, D. U. K. (2018); significant difference in parental occupation was seen in terms of social networking addiction.

5.2 REASONS FOR SOCIAL NETWORKING

Out of the 840 adolescents, the mean value of reasons for social networking was noted highest in fear on face to face interaction - 3.51 with the corresponding standard deviation 1.17. Reasons for social networking mean value was more for "I feel anxious, when the network is not available" -3.95 with the corresponding standard deviation 1.18. Correlation analysis finding suggest positive correlation between reasons for social networking and addiction whereas; negative correlation with mental health.

5.2.1 9 A's as Reasons for Social Networking

Adolescents in the present study accepted that there are various reasons for social networking. Affordability, Accessibility, Anonymity, Approximation, Ambiguity, Acceptability, and Accommodation are the7A's proposed by Hertlein & Stevenson (2010); that act as reasons for social networking. In addition to these, autonomy and availability are the two other A's that favors social networking; proved in this study.

Affordability compels the adolescents to use internet and its applications more, as social networking is cheap and easy to use (Chukwuere and Onyebukwa, 2017). These findings support the present research, as many of the adolescents engaged in social networking because it is affordable.

The increased accessibility has changed the pattern of internet use in the world (Cooper, 2000). Reasons for social networking also include free access (Young & Rogers, 1998). Anxiety was observed by Rosen et al (2013), when the adolescents were not able to access social networking sites. This feature can lead to addiction; Kuss, D. J., & Griffiths, M. D. (2011) stated that easy access favours addiction.

Social networking increases one's ability to promote chosen identity (Hertlein & Sendak, 2007). Anonymity is explicit in cyber-sex. McFarlane et al (2000) found that anonymity helped in having more partners; leads to a hike in sexually transmitted diseases (Bolding et al 2007). Thus it is clearer that through social networking privacy is maintained (Lennon et al 2012).

Approximation was originally added by Ross (2002) and Cooper et al (2003) regarding online sex. In this context, the quality of approximation of the internet is used as a stress and conflict management tool; it simulates a way to manage stress through sexual activity (Cooper et al 2004).

In the present study many adolescents agreed the fact that ambiguity is an influencing factor, when ambiguity increases, addictive tendency also increases. Social networking paved the way for faithful relationship; social networking can be ambiguous (Parker and Wampler, 2003).

The wide acceptance promotes social networking. Many students accept internet as a knowledge acquisition medium which is far better and greater than the traditional class room learning. (Cooper et al 2004) confirmed that social networking can be used to access sexual topics and is considered as acceptable.

The meaning of accommodation is that those individuals who have more difficulty settling the tension between the "real" versus "ought" self (Higgins, 1987) will be more likely to be taking risks on the internet, thus making their relationship vulnerable to affairs than those who do not. More evidence of the concept of accommodation is found in the research conducted by Aviram and Amichai-Hamburger (2005).

Because of amplified autonomy, adolescents may connect further in social networking and this propensity can end up in addiction. As per UNESCO, one can develop through internet. It provides an unprecedented volume of resources for information that opens up new opportunities, because of its privacy people engage more and more in social networking.

Now, internet connection is available in even remote areas, freely available in public places. With the introduction and availability of free data packages, addiction increased (Marahatta et al 2015). Thus it is evident that these reasons increase the engagement in social networking, in turn increases the chance of addiction.

5.2.2 Smart Phone as a Reason for Social Networking

One of the major reasons that have increased the growth of social networking is the increased interest in using smart phone. Among the 840 adolescents, the most used device to engage in social networking is smart phone and the least preferred device is mobile devices like Symbian phones. In 2014, 1.85 billion people were using smart phone and 2087 billion in 2020 (Holst 2019). The amount of time spent on smart phone increased by 35% in 2015 from 2014 (Newman et al 2015); in turn will increase social networking. The popular activity on smart phone is engaging in social networking (Nearly 80). As per Lenhart (2015), 15 to 17 year old adolescents own a smart phone; 68% of 13 and 14 year old own a smart phone. Smart phones provide a sense of comfort to its users; user friendly (Melumad et al 2015). Smart phones paved the way to susceptible increase in the use of mobile phones (Jeong et al 2016; Lee 2015). Smart phone can be used for various purposes like receiving calls, reading texts, emails, to download and to watch movies etc. (Vincent & Haddon 2017).

Raj et al (2018) found that 75.7% adolescents accessed social networking with the help of smart phone, thus making smart phone the most common gadget among the 388 adolescents. MMIN (2017) noticed that out of the 72% female hostellers, 48.55% engage in social networking. A sense of virtual community is fostered because of the social networking sites; (Chen and Lin, 2014), this attracts adolescents towards social networking. Adolescents engage in social networking more (Espinoza and Juvonen, 2011), they spent more time online using mobile phone to access internet and 97% of the adolescents own a mobile phone of which 64% are capable of using social networking (Nielsen, 2010). Adolescents who are using smart phones informed that they may not be able to live without it (Wajcman et al 2007). This can lead to addiction and it is negatively correlated with academic performance (Baert et al 2019), positively associated with psychological impact (Beranuy et al 2009); anxiety, insomnia (Jenaro et al 2007); features of decreased mental health (Babadi-Akashe et al 2014). Deyan (2019) reported that 66% of smart phone users showed signs of nomophobia, 71% keep their phones next to them or sleep with the phone and 75% use it in toilet; smart phone use and depression are correlated.

5.2.3 Parental Factors as Reasons for Social Networking

A risk taking behavior can be avoided through monitoring by parents as per Pujazon-Zazik (2010). Lack of parental control (Young and Rogers 1998) and less protective parents (Chen et al 2015) is another reason for increased social networking. Family atmosphere also contribute to the type of activity they chose in social networking (Wellman et al 2008), hence positive parenting and family-related factors prevent an adolescent from increased engagement in social networking (Van den Eijnden et al 2010).

5.2.4 Friends as a Reason for Social Networking

Irfan (2015) revealed that out of the 168 students, 67% started engaging in social networking because of peer pressure. Adolescents engage in social networking for companionship (Young & Rogers, 1998). Positive peer influences (Mohr & Rosén, 2017) and contact with prosocial adults outside the family context (Woolley & Grogan 2006) helps in reducing harmful behavior during adolescent period. Thus good friendship will promote healthy behavior, bad companionship can increase harmful behaviors, increased social networking addiction and even they can land up with other addictions eg: substance abuse.

5.2.5 Other Reasons for Social Networking

The other reasons for social networking stated by the adolescents in this study are in order to escape from studies, due to lack of life satisfaction, to reduce suicidal thoughts, because of fear on face to face interaction, to reduce stress, to reduce nervousness, because of excessive web surfing tendencies, interest in sending threatening email to frighten others and increased interest in online sex.

5.2.6 Escape from Studies, Forget Previous Bad Experiences

The life of students is full of stress as they have lot of school work, assignments, exams (Tandoc et al 2015); moreover adolescence is a period where there can be negative thoughts / feelings, state of apprehension and they use various defense mechanisms in order to escape from the situation. Caplan (2010); Giannakos (2013) stated that adolescents engage in social networking to escape from negative feelings and anxiety situations. They consider social networking as a means to escape from the negative feelings, when they feel burn out they engage more and more in social networking, usually to play online games and there by become addicts. Some spend leisure time without any activities, they will be feeling lonely and they might want to reveal their self / identity; hence prefer social networking (Arnett, 2007); offer opportunity to forget previous bad experience.

5.2.7 Lack of Life Satisfaction

Kross et al (2013) informed that lack of life satisfaction is noted in social networking users. People who have increased close relationships tend to have increased level of life satisfaction (Reis & Gable, 2003). Social relationship can even predict mental and physical health (Cohen 2004). Thus it can be concluded that adolescents who lack life satisfaction get immersed in social networking, boosts the relationship with others and this in turn increases life satisfaction. Life satisfaction is a predictor of social networking addiction (Bozoglan et al 2013); poor self-worth is seen in addiction. (Chan 2014) found connection between personality and life satisfaction.

5.2.8 Reduce Suicidal Thoughts, Stress and Nervousness

Berryman et al (2018) highlighted that adolescents express suicidal ideation through social networking. People with low self esteem tend to engage more in social networking to increase their self-image, self-esteem and confidence (Hawi and Samaha, 2019); this further reduces suicidal ideations. According to Kim et al (2009), in order to relieve loneliness and depression, one engages in social networking. This will elevate the mood, increases positive feeling and reduces suicidal thoughts.

Adolescents engage in social networking in order to escape from stress (Young & Rogers, 1998) and from difficult life experiences (Pomfret 2019). Stress and anxiety is alleviated through social networking (Aksoy et al 2013). An adolescent with social anxiety or depression can overcome these problems; reduce their stress level through virtual interactions (McKenna & Bargh 1998, 1999). The present study showed that nervousness is prevalent in some adolescents and they engage in social networking to reduce it. Adolescents might turn to social networking, to voice their support and frustration (Ball - Rokeach & DeFleur, 1976).

5.2.9 Fear On Face To Face Interaction

Escape from fear on face to face interactions is possible through social networking, a place where people can simply observe without any conversations; thereby they fulfill the component of escape (Ball-Rokeach, & DeFleur, 1976). Adolescents who are anxious or shy in face to face interaction also prefer social networking (Van Zalk & Tillfors 2017). The present study finding is related to these statements; the adolescents who had fear on face to face interaction preferred social networking in order to escape from the real world.

5.2.10 Excessive Web Surfing Tendencies

Surfing excessively; lead to distrust and suspicion among users, some may even look into others life- "creeping", for this reason they might engage unnecessarily in social networking (Bjornsen, 2018). This can further lead to various issues.

5.2.11 Interest in Sending Threatening e-mail to Frighten Others and Online Sex

Adolescents opt cyberbullying because of its anonymity; anonymous postings reported a notable amount of offensive posts (Black et al 2016). For the purpose of sexual exploration they engage in social networking (Adu-Kumi, 2016), the most frequently searched topic on internet is sex (Freeman – Longo and Blachard, 1998). Sexual satisfaction is achieved through erotic photos, sex videos and live sex acts (Cooper et al 2002). Cyber bullying is common among adolescents, can cause depression, anxiety (Younes et al 2016) and suicide (O'Keeffe & Clarke-Pearson 2011). (Young & DeAbreu, 2011) support these facts by stating that because of sending unwanted mails and online sex, internet is misused.

5.2.12 Purpose of Social Networking

While concerned with the purpose of social networking, the mean value was highest for entertainment -3.51 with the corresponding standard deviation -1.29; this was also proved by Khan (2017), adolescents commonly engage in social networking for entertainment. The other purposes of engaging in social networking by the adolescents in this study are to interact, to establish / maintain relationship with others, to increase the knowledge, to have entertainment and for online purchase.

The purpose of social networking is to have fun (Brandtzæg & Heim 2009; Ifinedo, 2016); to gain information academically (Aillere & McNicol 2018); learning (Benson and Morgan, 2016); in order to stay in touch (Sharma & Shukla 2016); to connect (Livingstone, 1998; Salehan et al 2017); to boost up the older relations (Lampe et al 2007); to form identity, for rapport, increased social life (Ifinedo, 2016) and for communication (Matthews – Juarez et al 2013; Turner 2015; Phua et al 2017). Online friends are an integral part of teen social network (Lenhart et al 2015), to send message and meet friends one engage in social networking (Mohamed and Sumitha, 2011; Sardar, 2012). As per Kim et al 2010, social networking is used to share various content such as blogs, videos and photos to stay connected and to find new friends. Adolescents also engage in social networking in order to collect information about shops, brands and to purchase (Barnes et al 2008). Because of these reasons adolescents engage in social networking and can lead to too much of use and addiction (Cabral 2008).

5.3 SOCIAL NETWORKING IMPACTS

The extent of impact revealed the influence of social networking. This is related to addiction and mental health. Correlation analysis in this study proved negative correlation between mental health and physical, academic, psychological, adjustment and familial impacts; whereas there exists a significant positive correlation between social networking addiction and these impacts. Multiple regression proved relationship between social networking impacts and addiction, mental health. Confirmatory factor analysis proved that the impact that influences mental health the most is psychological impact. Social networking addiction can lead to various physical and mental health impacts (Young K 1998; Rosen et al 2013; Andreassen 2015). Thus it is evident that adolescents face awfully relentless impacts in their day to day life, because of the increased engagement in social networking (Young, 2004).

5.3.1 Physical Impacts

The study finding pointed that when there is social networking addiction, there will be physical problems and as the intensity of addiction increases, mental health deteriorates and the problems related to physical health increases. This finding is correlating with the definition of health by the WHO (Callahan 1973). The major finding which is noted in physical impacts is that nearly half of the adolescents reported that they have reduced sleep. Sleep is related to both physical and mental health. Adolescent health is determined by night time sleep (Woods & Scott, 2016). Decreased quality of sleep is found due to increased social networking (Cramer, 2018) and this can affect the health. As good sleep is essential to good mental health (Robotham, 2011), decreased sleep will direct to poor mental health; this will make people less receptive to positive emotions, sadness (Woodson, 2005). Sleep will have further impact in academics, psychological areas also. Head ache, muscle pain, irritation in eyes, bone problems are the other physical impacts due to social networking (Young K 1998; Rosen et al 2013; Andreassen 2015; Li et al 2018).

5.3.2 Academic Impacts

As it was noted in this study, Kubey et al (2001) also found positive correlation between social networking addiction and academic impact. Negative correlation between academic impact and mental health was also evident in this study. Decreased academic performance (Young, 1996, 1998), academic failure (Holtz & Appel, 2011) occur in social networking; poor academic performance occur due to the addiction in social networking (Young K 1998; Rosen et al 2013; Ahad & Lim, 2014; Andreassen 2015; Heffner 2016). According to Naizabekov (2012), students will keep their work in pending due to social networking. The grades are affected negatively due to procrastination and reading unnecessary stuff on social networking (Jacobsen and Forste, 2011). Adolescents will switch from one activity to another in social networking (Kirschner and Karpinski, 2010), this behavior can reduce the academic performance (Rosen et al 2013). As per Ahmadi and Zeinali (2018) social networking reduces the quality of sleep and increases academic stress; Gabre and Kumar (2012) found that social networking can cause stress and this stress will affect the academic achievement. Bijari et al (2013) stated that increased time spent in social networking will cause tiredness, poor sleep and this will lead to poor concentration and learning. Thus the other impacts of social networking has an influence; directly or indirectly in academic performance.

If the adolescent engage in social networking in a productive manner it leads to positive impacts; practical knowledge increases (Akakandelwa and Walubita 2018), social networking smoothens school work, knowledge sharing and collaboration occurs between friends in social networking. Bardakci et al (2018) stated that students interact with their classmates and teachers through social networking; this will enhance social interaction and learning. A study by Tuan & Tu (2013) has proved that social networking improved the performance / grade of students. Thus it is obvious that if the adolescents engage in social networking for a prolonged time, it can cause addiction and affect the academics negatively; if they use social networking for knowledge gain and in a limited amount, it will increase the academic performance (Heffner 2016).

5.3.3 Psychological Impacts

Features of depression, anxiety and reduced subjective wellbeing are noted among adolescents who spent more time in social networking (Primack et al 2017); cling to the findings of the present study. Increased social networking results in social networking addiction that consecutively results in anxiety and depression (Young & Rogers, 1998; Rosen et al 2013; Andreassen 2015; Younes et al 2016; Primack et al 2017); as well as psychological dependence and behavioral issues (Gámez-Guadix et al 2013; Gámez-Guadix et al 2014). Social networking has positive effects on psychological wellbeing (Kraut 1998), reduced loneliness, increased happiness and well-being (Young, 1997; Ellison et al 2007), obtained through the limited use.

5.3.4 Adjustment Impacts

From the correlation analysis it is unmistakable that when the mental health reduces, adjustment also will be poor. When there is social networking addiction, the adolescent will have poor adjustment and poor mental health. Adjustment is a basic quality / characteristic feature of mental health, an adolescent who is mentally healthy will adjust with others; conflict and aggressive behavior arises when there is no adjustment. As connectedness and happiness is improved through social networking (Valkenburg et al 2006); it can promote the adjustment quality, if the adolescent engage in it without getting addicted.

5.3.5 Familial Impacts

If the adolescent is frequently engaged in social networking, he / she may not be interested in family and problems arise. Thus social networking addiction is a cause at the rear of family issues (Young K 1998; Rosen et al 2013; Andreassen 2015). Even though social networking increases family ties, connections and relationships; it has to be used appropriately, sensitively and has to be managed effectively. Otherwise adolescents can get addicted and negative impacts can arise.

5.4 SOCIAL NETWORKING AND MENTAL HEALTH

Social networking has become an indispensable part of day today life and almost all adolescents engross in it. Frequency analysis was done to assess the extent of social networking that result in addictive pattern. The results showed that 63.8% of the adolescents (n=536) engage in social networking without any addiction; whereas 28.9% (n=243) were addicted mildly; 5.6 % (n=47) moderately and only 1.7% (n=14) were severely addicted. This finding is similar to the study by Akakandelwa & Walubita (2017), showed decreased social networking addiction. That is, among the 240 students, 13.7% strongly disagreed that they are addicted, 29.5% disagreed, 34.4% reported neutral, 17.6% agreed and 4.8% strongly agreed that they feel like addicted in social networking. Correlation analysis revealed positive relationship between reasons and impacts of social networking with addiction. Multiple regression proved relationship between social networking impacts and addiction.

Emotional dependence on the internet is termed as addiction (Jonathan, 1998). The difference between excessive engagement in social networking and social networking addiction is that the latter is associated with unfavorable impacts when online, becomes uncontrollable and compulsive (Andreassen, 2015). It is evident that majority of the students in this study were not having compulsive behavior. Social networking addiction is one type of behavioral addiction and it reflects problematic engagement in it (Andreassen, 2015; Shensa et al 2017; Bjornsen, 2018). Features of social networking addiction include tolerance, withdrawal problems, conflict, salience, relapse, and mood modification (Andreassen, 2015); changes in mood, not interested in work / self care, withdrawal symptoms, preoccupation with social networking, not able to cut down usage and psychological issues (Tang and Koh 2019). There will be repetitive, uncontrollable thoughts related to social networking (Bjornsen, 2018) among the addicted ones; these features are suggestive of addiction-related behaviors (Sultan et al 2014).

The positive and negative influence was identified on the basis of addiction – non addiction criteria; increased addiction projects the dark side and absence of addiction indicates healthy use. The positive impacts of social networking are the high light of this study. Various benefits are associated with social networking; education, supportive relationship, identity formation, increased sense of belonging and adaptation in stressful circumstances (Third et al 2011). The adolescents in this study (63.8%) are engaging in social networking in a prolific way, devoid of reaching in to addiction. This is reliable with the statement-through social networking people communicate with others in several ways without getting addicted (Nielson, 2012).

In order to recognize the extent of mental health among social networking users, frequency analysis was done and the result showed that among the adolescents, 53.9% (n=453) were found to have low mental health and 46.1% (n=387) were having high mental health. Correlation analysis proved negative correlation between reasons, social networking impacts, addiction and mental health. Multiple regression revealed relationship between social networking impacts and mental health. Social networking has an impact on mental health (Valkenburg et al 2006; Kross et al 2013; Verduyn et al 2015).

The study clearly indicates that social networking has to be used only in a controlled way; it may increase the mental health if used properly. Even though some adolescents are having low mental health, social networking can enhance their psychological wellbeing (Gross et al 2002; Campbell, 2005; Boase et al 2006; Burns et al 2007; Burns et al 2009). This is comparable to the notion, (Aksoy et al 2013) stress and anxiety is alleviated through social networking. Resilience is promoted through social networking; thus, it helps in adapting to the stressful event and the change in life (Oliver et al 2006).

Excessive social networking predict poor mental health (Ciarrochi et al 2016). Frequent engagement in social networking does not necessarily indicate addiction (Griffiths, 2010); therefore, does not always have negative impacts on mental health (Pasek & Hargittai, 2009; Jelenchick et al 2013). It can harm the client by reducing the mental health in case of improper, excessive use. Thus etiology behind poor mental health is social networking addiction. Reduced mental health can in turn increase the social networking penchant and vice versa. Caplan (2005) considered low psychological well-being as the cause and the effect of virtual addiction. Adolescents with social networking addiction will have negative impacts and there by low mental health. This quintessence of the present study upshot is supported by Rosen et al (2012). The adolescents in this study revealed that they need more time for social networking; but greater screen time (Gupta et al 2018) and continuous availability online (Krishnamurthy & Chetlapalli, 2015) can cause social networking addiction. This highlights that there exists a relationship between the time spent online and mental health (Gámez-Guadix, 2014).

The structural equation model also revealed that social networking impacts have a positive influence on addiction and addiction influences mental health negatively. This is in line with the conceptual model; emphasize on primary prevention, that is early detection of features and prevention of mental illness. When the negative impacts of social networking increases, chances of addiction also increases. The adolescents exhibit features of addiction, that include tolerance, dependence, withdrawal issues, negative impacts and craving towards social networking. In case of addicted adolescents, positive mental wellbeing starts reducing and the adolescent will deviate from the normal mental health. Once the mental health issues are not taken care of properly the mental health further deteriorates and the features of mental illness can develop.

5.5 QUALITATIVE ANALYSIS

In order to explore more on the social networking impacts, qualitative study was done and this made the study an in depth one. The quantitative analysis revealed that the negative impacts can deteriorate mental health. The main purpose of qualitative analysis in this study is to recognize the bright side of social networking and in fact comprehend the adolescent social networking behavior. The final triangulation of data helped to enrich and contextualize the finding. The diagrammatic representation of the process followed is given below.

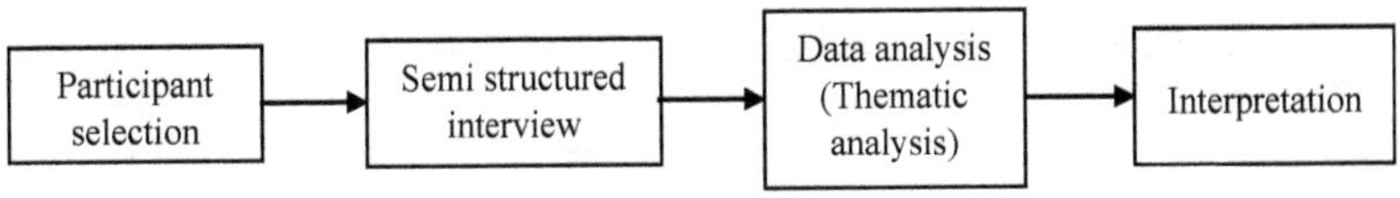

Four participants were selected for the study, one from each category of social networking addiction (No addiction, mild, moderate, and severe addiction). Confidentiality was maintained, the participants preferred to be kept anonymous. The verbal and nonverbal contents were transcribed for further analysis. The present section deals with the results of the analysis of qualitative data obtained through the in-depth interviews conducted with the chosen adolescents.

According to Braun and Clarke (2006), thematic analysis comprises of identification, analysis and the reporting of patterns occurring within the obtained data. It includes a set of definite stages beginning with familiarization with the data through systematic reading and comprehension of the obtained raw data. The next stage involves generation of initial codes which refer to meaningful items within the data that seem to recur. Subsequently sorting and organizing the obtained codes into potential themes is carried out. During the following stage the themes are revised by thorough examination of both the codes as well as the potential themes arrived at. Defining and naming the final themes based upon the nature of the themes is the second last step. The concluding stage includes production of the report of the analysis thus conducted.

5.5.1 Theme Generation

The verbatim responses of the participants were categorized into themes. In the initial stage of theme generation, identification of themes is outlined based on codes and categories. Firstly, themes were identified by outlining connections within and between participants, categories, and codes. For gathering detailed information regarding the purpose, thoughts, feelings, impacts, consequences, and problems related to social networking open ended questions was asked and semi structured interview was carried out.

5.5.2 Research Questions

1. What is the purpose of social networking?
2. What are the thoughts that emerge when engaged in social networking?
3. What are the feelings (emotions) when engaged in social networking?
4. What are the impacts of social networking?
5. How social networking affects personal, academic and social life?
6. Is social networking a healthy behavior?

The present section deals with the results of the analysis of qualitative data obtained through the in-depth interviews conducted with the chosen respondents. Thematic analysis was done to explore answers for the questions asked and the details are given below:

1. What is the purpose of social networking?

Participant 1: "Initially I used to watch movies; search Google for my study purpose, when I feel sad, when I am alone smart phone is my friend. I can chat with others". "I have private chats even old ladies and strangers come and join with me, I used to spend my leisure hours and evening in chatting. When I chat with my friends, I forget my worries, feel happy, feel comfortable and more confident, now I can't live without chatting, use to watch porn videos, movies, sexual chats and I enjoy it, get relief, satisfaction though this".

Participant 2: "I was very happy to chat with, in order to show that I have many friends, I keep on adding friends, I chat with many boys. I will be online whole night, feel relaxed, burn out feeling will be gone". "I used to get suicidal thoughts, want to get rid of my life. When this thought arises, I chat with friends and I get relief." I even mingle with strangers through WhatsApp and Facebook". I am happy to see them and talk to them through IMO, SKYPE, WhatsApp, I check timeline messages, add selfie, share blog, troll; use Twitter, add photos in Instagram. Now it is a hobby for me and

I enjoy my life only because of this, as I can contact my friends. I chat with friends, have sexual talks, download videos, movies songs and used to watch.

Participant 3: "Day time I used to mingle with friends in the school can't see them during night time, so I make contact with them through video call." At first, I used to prepare my project with the help of YouTube, search google for study purpose and later on started calling friends, play online games, I felt happy after this, it's a superb experience".

Participant 4: "I used to chat whole night and watch sex videos from various sites like stripchat.com, xvideos.com etc. I used to download nude photos of film stars and sex videos". "Yes I always chat with my friends, sometimes I use it for writing assignments, as it gives me an easy access to the information that I need. When I am free I watch movies and videos, it gives happiness to me". "Many times, I get involved in WhatsApp as it is a time pass to me. Among our friends we used to share photos and videos online and we find a good time to discuss about it while we meet". "Whenever I feel like talking to my friends, it's always helpful to have a Smartphone with good internet connection, so that I can communicate quickly and freely without any delay". I order foods, book tickets online".

2. What are the thoughts that emerge when engaged in social networking?

Participant 1: "I think of meeting people whom I chat, think of purchasing fashionable clothes online, I want to be online always, time is not enough, I need more time".

Participant 2: "When I am online, I like to have sexual talks with others, I enjoy it and these kinds of thoughts come to my mind".

Participant 3: "No specific thoughts arise when online, but I often think on the basis of what I am going online". "When not using net, thoughts of using WhatsApp arise and I think about what I have done before and I again use it. I think that using social networking is having merits and disadvantages, it is a very good thing to reduce boring.

When I am not online, I think about using it, can't think of a world without WhatsApp, I think that it's a precious gift of technology".

Participant 4: "When I open WhatsApp, I see others online and I chat with them, make video calls, then I think of going to Facebook and then again to WhatsApp".

3. What are the feelings (emotions) when engaged in social networking?

Participant 1: "I feel happy and I get so much of relief, I feel refreshed". "I feel energetic and hopeful about my life, when I think about being online. It offers a lot of information regarding everything I need and I am highly satisfied about this".

Participant 2: "I feel crazy to chat; everyone should feel the thrill of chatting". "It makes me relaxed," "I feel comfortable". "When I chat with my friends, I feel very happy and when we continue sharing our ideas it's actually a fun time for us".

Participant 3: "I feel angry when I am not able to use WhatsApp or Facebook, I get irritated when someone disturbs my personal time with my Smartphone, I feel like killing those who intervene when I chat with my close friends, it gives me a "Wow" feeling, I feel like the whole world is within my reach".

Participant 4: "I feel very cheerful and my mind becomes calm and pleasant when using WhatsApp, Facebook".

4. What are the impacts of social networking?

Participant 1: "Yes of course, it helps in mingling with friends, to keep in touch with them, it is helpful to pass time, reduces boring, I prefer Google, it gives lot of information, latest news, we can increase our knowledge, download books and can join online learning. It reduces our heaviness of mind; it is a friend, when I am alone". "Yes, I think that social media is a necessity, I can't avoid that, it helps in faster and direct communication. It gives lots of information, helps me relax, you can reach anywhere and search for anything, we will get it". "I search Google for my study purpose, watch movies". "I chat with my friends".

Participant 2: "I am here because of my WhatsApp, Facebook friends. They used to console me when I chat with them. I get lot of relief through chatting. It is a time pass for me. When I am immersed online, I forget all my worries, thoughts. I think of living and I feel charm, relaxed during chatting. It reduces my pressure and heaviness of chest. At night, when I am not able to sleep, I feel relaxed because of chatting, video call".

Participant 3: "My boy friend's will chat with me every day, keep contact with them through video call and engage in online games. I search Google for study purpose, prepares project with the help of YouTube, send photos and songs to friends".

Participant 4: "I get more than what I get from class; I can learn whenever I get time, it's more informative, watching Youtube videos related to my studies help me to learn more, I get more detailed information about my interest- areas, I also chat with students from other countries, it encourages learning".

5. Is social networking a healthy behavior?

Participant 1: "I don't think that there are any problems in using social media, I am capable of using it whenever I want it and can engage in my studies well".

Participant 2: "The world is changing; this is needed in everyone's life".

Participant 3: "I used to prepare my projects with the help of Youtube. I search Google for study purpose, it's a superb experience".

Participant 4: "Yes, everybody needs to use it. It's always good, I can't live without it".

6. What are the problems faced due to social networking?

Participant 1: "I get immersed in it and sometimes sit for hours without moving out... I often feel sleepy during daytime, many times I get scolded by my parents and even though I know that I am using it for long hours, I am not able to resist its use. I feel headache after long hours of using it and often have the pain in my hands, neck, and shoulder regions".

Participant 2: "I am not interested in studies, I feel tired and sleepy during day times, every time I check my phone for message. Again and again I check my phone and if my friends are not there, I feel sad, frustrated. If my mother talks to me, when I am online I feel irritated".

Participant 3: "I feel tired and sleepy during day time. Sometimes I hear ringtones of mobile phone / voices when I am sitting alone. I used to go to church every day, but now I won't get up in the morning and so can't attend the holy mass. My parents quarrel with e because I won't get up as usual; sometimes I will be with mobile phone and didn't even eat food, not opening my books".

Participant 4: "I need to open WhatsApp and see the messages as soon as I open my eyes, I will be online throughout the day. I used to hear music before, but now my hobby is chatting. Sometimes, I forget to take bath, whole night I will be with WhatsApp and Facebook. Morning I feel sleepy, used to get headache, feel irritated at times when people ask about my studies. If I sit alone, I think of using WhatsApp, Facebook and I want to spend more time in it. Many times, I heard ringing mobile phones even though it was not".

Qualitative analysis with the help of semi structured interview, open ended questions revealed the facts and hidden ideas about social networking among the adolescents. Social networking was unavoidable among them, used it for various reasons and it has had both positive and negative impacts. The adolescents were more curious and happy about the bright side of social networking; benefits include connectedness, positive emotions, privacy, independency, need satisfaction and feeling of togetherness. The adolescents informed that they can get whatever they want through social networking, things can be purchased without moving out from the house, it saves time, energy and money. According to the adolescents, social networking is a healthy behavior; they are not aware of the consequences hidden in it. Initially they started engaging in social networking for academic purpose and then started exploring it. Many of the adolescents were stressed and in order to reduce tension they engaged in social networking. As they are the vulnerable group, there is more chances of deviating from normality and due to this tendencies for increased social networking can occur. Increased social networking will suppress the positive impacts and negative impacts can project. Those who deviated from the productive use experienced various physical, academic, psychological, adjustment and familial problems. Because of the poor sleep, they could not concentrate in the class and landed up in poor academic performance. Excessive engagement can lead to negative impacts, addiction and this can deteriorate mental health; mental illness can occur. Thus the qualitative study concludes that social networking enhances mental health, if it is used in an appropriate manner otherwise negative impacts can arise and the adolescents can land up in addiction and poor mental health.

5.6 IMPLICATIONS OF THE STUDY

The study on "The Influence of Social Networking on Mental Health" reveals that social networking is having a positive and negative impact. The adolescents in this study had negative impacts in physical, academic, psychological, adjustment and familial areas. The adolescents may be unaware of the negative impacts; instructions on enhancing student's academic proficiency and there by shift their attention productively to use social networking applications has to be promoted. If the students engage in social networking when they feel exhausted, bored or stressed up, they feel relaxed and after that they should be offline and should concentrate in their studies. Parental monitoring is needed for this. During the study time, if they get doubts, they can very well utilize social networking, can clarify doubts. Their knowledge can be improved through social networking; relationship can be enhanced, and can even achieve positive emotions through fun. Sessions on the healthy use of social networking will enhance positive impacts whereas awareness about the dark side will reduce negative impacts.

Many adolescents engage in social networking for their sexual desires, and knowingly or unknowingly become addicts; social networking is a joyful addiction. The usage should be restricted by keeping monitoring measures and sources to protect them from committing cybercrimes or falling into traps hidden in the cyber world. The issue of social networking addiction is important to consider because as electronic revolutions become not just tools but essential aspects of our lives, use and misuse can happen.

Though the extensive criteria of social networking addiction is not yet definitive, the present study reveals the fact that social networking addiction exists among adolescents and is a significant problem that requires the attention of mental health professionals, educationalists and parents. Furthermore, professionals in education sector need to be aware of preventing, identifying and handling the adolescents vulnerable to social networking addiction. Thus the study highlights the necessity for parental supervision and to educate the adolescents regarding the dark side of social networking.

5.7 RECOMMENDATIONS

Measures should be initiated to increase the mental health of the adolescents. Detailed in depth counseling should be conducted to at risk students. Focus has to be given on primary prevention. Mental health camps can be conducted in the schools by the mental health professionals in order to identify features of addiction, mental illness. Sessions on characteristics of mental health, mental illness has to be taken to the students and parents.

The education department should include the bright and dark side of social networking in the curriculum, new policies, separate platform for students can be introduced. The study calls for a vigilant responsiveness on the part of respective authorities including school and family to take necessary steps to prevent adolescents from being lost in the world of social networking. Schools should maintain firm rules and regulations to prevent problematic social networking. Unwanted sites should be prohibited to the students. Strict parental monitoring and time limit has to be set in adolescent's social networking. Inputs on merits and demerits of social networking can be provided to the students and parents in meetings. Schools can tie up with service organisations offering 24 hours counselling, for the benefits of students and parents. Various therapies can be provided in the schools, if not available. Leisure time activities, hobbies should be nurtured in order to divert from stress and social networking. Instead of leaning to social networking for fun, outdoor and indoor games has to be promoted.

5.8 LIMITATIONS

It was difficult for the researcher to get adequate support from the school authorities, as they were more focussed on student's education. The researcher covered only limited number of schools due to the time constraint. After the study, further intervention based on the results such as implementation of therapies was not done due to the time constraint. Some parents were more concerned with the children's education rather than mental health, did not give consent for the study. Even though features of mental illness were identified, could not diagnose it because of the non-availability of psychiatrist in schools.

5.9 SCOPE FOR FUTURE RESEARCH

- Further research is required to find ways to prevent the student community from falling into the virtual trenches in the vast ocean of social networking, that are dangerous to physical, psychological and social functioning.

- Exclusive research can be done on various social media applications separately and its influence on mental health can be explored.

- Comparative study between early, late and middle adolescents can be conducted.

- Similar study can be conducted in different settings such as primary schools, colleges and other higher educational institutions.

- Social networking usage in pandemics can be evaluated.

- Qualitative studies among adolescents should be increased as the in-depth interviews will reveal the hidden areas associated with the aetiology behind social networking.

- Qualitative studies can be imparted among parents to explore the reasons and factors behind the adolescent's social networking.

- Social networking among the employed and unemployed can be surveyed.

- Mental health professionals should conduct studies in each school, to assess the online behavior.

5.11 CONCLUSION

The study finding proved that as the reasons for social networking increases, the social networking addiction also increases. When the social networking impacts and addiction increases, the mental health reduces. In fact, the over-engagement of social networking will result in physical problems, problems related to education, psychological problems and issues in family relationships. As far as the impact of social networking is concerned, the most influential impact on mental health is psychological impact; where as physical impacts are influencing addiction the most. Social networking is not self-destructive on its own, but to a certain extent it is the way of using it that leads to consequences. The appropriate use of social networking requires a background and responsiveness of how they should be used exactly in a right way. Even though only few adolescents in this study were severely addicted, there is chance for others to become addicts in the future. The non addicts will be utilizing the bright side of social networking, but increased use can further lead to negative impacts. In this regard, the results of the study indicate the need for motivation to the students by parents and teachers in the social networking area, to help them to engage in social networking in a productive manner. If the use of social networking is managed properly, it will increase the productivity; if not, increased negative consequences arise at the individual and social level. Moreover, the mental health will get sapped due to addiction; if this is not managed properly features of mental illness can ascend. Thus the study also climaxes social networking addiction as one of the major etiology behind poor mental health. As the adolescents are the looming populaces, if the mental health is not preserved they will not be able to accomplish academic heights and will not be able to lead a worthy fruitful life.

CPSIA information can be obtained
at www.ICGtesting.com
Printed in the USA
LVHW022046140423
744403LV00010B/454

9 784759 188264